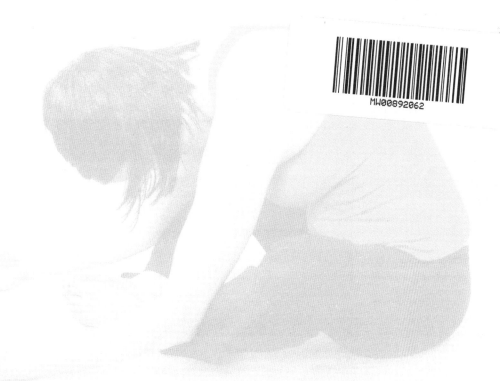

LETTING GO
roll & relax into release

by Bella Dreizler
physical therapist & yoga teacher

copyright 2011

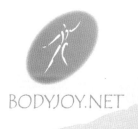

BODYJOY.NET

table of contents

introduction

Consider this fact: the more we inhabit our bodies, the easier it is for us to heal. This book is a practical guide to physical embodiment that blends time-tested physical therapy techniques and the cutting edge of yin yoga. Step into a world that will deepen your relationship with your body and amp up your internal knowledge of movement, breath and sensation.

Practices like yoga, dance and martial arts help us become more fully embodied. But sometimes we are sidelined by our injuries or stiffness. These challenges take us away from the very movement medicine we need. Vulnerability and fear can create paralyzing inertia. As the saying goes, sometimes the spirit is willing but the flesh is weak. The injuries that keep us from enjoying a physical practice are as varied as the bodies we inhabit: back problems, hip tightness, recurring foot issues, neck injuries, shoulder restrictions. The list goes on!

How to work with our unique body limitations is what this guide is all about. We'll discover, open and soften restrictions with physical therapy release tools: balls and rollers. We'll let new levels of flexibility flow right out of gentle yin yoga. We'll access new found internal support for posture and alignment. There is so much wisdom to gain from mindful movement and attunement to our precious body.

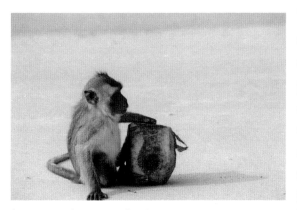 There is an old Chinese fable that details how to set a monkey trap: cut an opening in a coconut the size of a monkey's open hand, place some rice in the bottom of the hollow and place this fruit trap where the monkeys travel. When a curious monkey reaches in to grab the rice, his tight fisted hold will not fit back out through the opening. The lesson is obvious. Just like the monkey, we need to learn to let go of whatever our version of the rice happens to be. Learning to let go of the restrictions in our body often delivers us to a deeply personal meaning about what it is we need to release in our lives.

A conscious connection of the body to heart and mind can put us in touch with our authentic instincts, intuition and insight. When we trust our own movement, breath and sensation we are guided to the source of emotion, to our very soul and spirit. Investing time in a supportive practice like the one detailed in this book can be an end in itself, our own personal yoga. Regular commitment to these techniques will also pave the way to safe participation in other physical movement practices.

Let this book guide you to:

· explore your unique patterns of tightness

· develop expertise in targeting what structures need your time

· the correct, most effective use of the foam roller & balls to loosen short connective tissue

· correctly holding specific yin poses to lengthen connective tissue restrictions

· the bhandas: the yogic approach to functional core strength

· using breath and sensation so mindful meditation integrates the practice

Creatively make these techniques your own until you:

· become familiar with your body's normal patterns of asymmetry

· have a full healthy range of motion

· are less prone to injury and recover more quickly

· develop your intuitive muscle and become your own best body worker

Some of these activities may be contraindicated if, for example, you have osteoporosis, fractures, numb areas, open wounds and sensitive diabetes. Please consult your doctor before engaging in any of these practices if you have special concerns. This is a self-awareness practice. You must commit to monitoring your personal response to each exercise if this approach is to be successful for you.

Acknowledgements

I am grateful to the thousands of courageous patients who continue to let me into their lives, allowing me to coach and witness the unique unraveling of their challenges. Thank you to my students who patiently and regularly show up in class and help me know what works and what does not. Thank you to my many teachers in the world of orthopedic manual therapy and yoga. A particularly big hug to Sukbhir Collins, the former owner of Deep Yoga in Sacramento, my hometown. Blessings on Gabrielle Roth and my decade long immersion in 5Rhythms for the way it opened me to a wider world of possibility. Thank you to my husband Bob Dreizler for standing by me through all my unfolding and for being such an awesome photographer. Thank you to Cassie McCann who posed patiently for so many photos and thank you to Stacy Hayden for taking this raw material and turning it into a book. Thanks to my posse for standing around the kitchen one night and brainstorming the name for this book!

before you begin

Why do I need this?

As we age, stiffness and tightness in our body begins to feel like the new norm. Injuries, heredity, gravity, emotional patterns and postural habits contribute to this universal human condition. There are plenty of exercise practices that focus on muscles: how to strengthen them and how to stretch. When we're young, we can exercise muscles and boost power and flexibility with relative ease. As time marches on, the role of connective tissue and its effect on our flexibility becomes increasingly important.

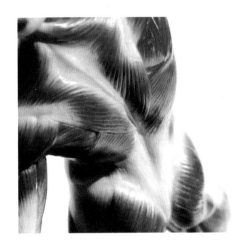

Connective tissue includes the bones and the cartilage, the tendons attaching muscle to bone, the ligaments binding bones together and the deep fascia that binds muscles together. Collagen fibers are the building blocks of connective tissue and are the root cause of ordinary stiffness. Injuries, habits and age change them from pliable and elastic to rusty, short and a bit deranged. As they tighten, they draw muscle and bone closer, creating less possibility for movement.

Much of our tightness develops in predictable asymmetrical patterns. For more than two decades I have been developing ways to help us break down collagen changes in connective tissue, especially tightness around the hips, spine and shoulders. This is the foundation of my individual client treatment and workshop instruction. After years of teaching group exercise classes in connection with clinical physical therapy work, I began to explore the vast world of yoga. For the last few years I have been drawn to yin yoga because of the way it effectively addresses this connective tissue concern.

We are living beings comprised of living tissues. When these tissues are stressed, they adapt and actually change. We already know about these kind of adaptive changes from our experience following an injury. We can feel tightness develop in response to a harmful stress. Less obvious are the restrictions that slowly develop over time because of the habitual ways we hold ourselves. However, stresses can be positive as well and can be applied in a purposefully therapeutic way. Connective tissue restrictions release when subjected to just the right amount of stress. Over and over again I have seen and experienced decreases in tightness with using the roller and balls and engaging in long-held yin poses.

What is the problem?

The curves in our spine provide us with balance and a central axis from which to move. There are two forward curves (neck and low back) and two backward curves (upper back and tail). Healthy curves have the capacity to move further into the direction they are headed and into the opposing direction as well. The spine moves in a twisting direction, too. Most of us lose mobility in the motions of these curves, each of us in our own unique way. Regaining motion takes awareness, commitment, and patience.

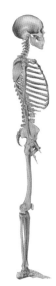

There are many patterns of movement loss. These are very common:

- Too much neck extension: unable to drop chin to chest or turn the head fully from side to side

- Too much upper back flexion: unable to lift breast bone or expand ribs; difficulty twisting side to side

- Fixed in slight low back flexion: unable to arch low back backward or bend it forward

When the spine becomes immobile, the shoulders and hips always follow. When a tight neck creates a forward head and a hunched upper back creates a caved-in breastbone, the shoulder joint becomes very unhappy. Irritation of the rotator cuff tendons is very common and often stems from this central issue. This can also be the root cause of tennis elbow, carpal tunnel syndrome and symptoms of numbness or tingling in the arms. Trying to "fix" only the shoulder or the elbow or the wrist without addressing the spinal inflexibility gets us nowhere fast.

Just as the shoulder cannot be separated from the upper back, the hips are intimately tied to the low back and sacroiliac joint. Hips are also linked to restrictions in all the tissues attaching below: hamstrings, psoas, adductors, rotators and iliotibial band. Most

9

of the ways we "open" the hips are in conjunction with opening all these other areas as well.

What is the solution?

Learning to effectively use the balls and rollers helps us to break up the connective tissue restrictions. Engaging in yin poses that address our personal restrictions will re-establish the length and pliability of the tissue.

Each of the target release areas have corresponding energy points in many other health education models. There are maps of meridians and chakras that guide many alternative practitioners. As you release, you will be affecting connective tissue right along with many of these lines and centers. It is not unusual to experience emotional responses during self-release work. We can learn to trust our breath to carry flashes of insight and emotion right through us as we find a way to work right on our edge.

Luckily learning how to release connective tissue does not require knowledge of these energetic systems or the structural names and function of the tissues. What we do need to know is how to make adjustments so that we feel release happening at our personal edge in the specific region we are targeting.

What is our personal edge?

Let's say it right here: breaking up tight collagen restrictions is usually uncomfortable. Creating discomfort is really scary for some of us but without some discomfort, nothing changes. Some people refer to this sensation as a "good hurt". Each of us must find our personal edge and remember that it varies from day to day. We know we have passed our edge and are in possible danger of making ourselves worse when we notice that we have stopped breathing and we are tensing in areas other than the target. On the flip side, we are not at our edge yet when there is no sensation created in the target. Lack of sensation means that nothing is being stressed for adaptive change in the tissue. This edge finding takes undivided self-focus and attention. This is not an activity to undertake while watching T.V. This is the very essence of a yoga practice: deep awareness of the breath, undivided attention on sensation, union of body and mind.

How do I know what to do?

The professional world of manual orthopedic physical therapy is simple and elegant, arising from the best of science. Patients come with specific body challenges. Together we review symptoms: how they began and how they behave. We look at active movement and the role of posture and alignment. Together we find movements that reliably re-create the pain. Specific hands on table work aims to manually release tight structures that might be creating the problem. Often the tightness is in a different area than the pain. When we are satisfied we have found the target or targets, we fine-tune the self-care.

We learn how to:

- Loosen what is tight with balls and rollers

- Lengthen what is short with yin yoga poses

- Stabilize what is weak with posture and alignment

I have worked with many students in classes and workshops who take on this process without individual professional guidance. This is totally possible if your body challenge is uncomplicated and you have solid body awareness. You can use this guide to explore all the typical tight regions on the human body and see what is true for you. Learning to release on your own is more complicated when you have multiple regions affected and if your symptoms radiate from the spine into the arms or legs. Seek the help of a qualified physical therapist if this applies to you.

How do I use the roller and balls?

Over the years I have experimented with many tools to reproduce what my hands do in treatment. The release techniques in this book rely on the use of these three tools:

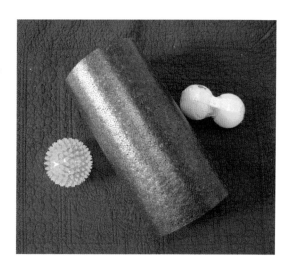

- *foam roller:* purchase a quality 6" wide roller that will not flatten with use. Use the 3 foot long one if you are large. The one foot version is enough for average size people and has the advantage of being portable, cheaper and less styrofoam.

- *pokey ball:* The search for perfection on this item has been a long time quest.

Look for a ball with hard enough spikes to bring you to an edge of discomfort. If you are lean and lanky, you may need to use something softer and spike-less like a single tennis or racquet ball.

• *double tennis balls:* Use filament embedded strapping tape to tightly wrap two new or used balls together: twice around the long way, twice around in between the balls.

You can visit www.bodyjoy.net/book.html for information on purchasing the foam roller and pokey ball.

The surface you choose to work on is important. There will be less pressure with a thick rug or mat and more pressure on a bare floor. Take time to accurately adjust your position so that you feel you are on the target area. Bring just the right pressure to bear for perfect delivery to your edge. Actively massage the region or rest into the unique spots that feel tightest. Use each exhale to visualize the area melting. Use as many breaths as needed to let go as fully as you are able.

When you find the perfect edge, there is sometimes a burning, hot sensation while pressure is applied and a flush of warmth and tingling on completion. Move the body in any way that feels intuitively right for release then take a rest and focus on the slow wane of sensation before coming into the next technique.

The techniques listed are simply a jumping off point for your own creative exploration. Cracking and popping of the joints are normal in the upper back. Repeatedly cracking the low back or neck has questionable value and may even be detrimental. Continually monitor the body for relaxation. These are some sure signs of tension, clues that you are working too aggressively: scrunching up the face, clenching the buttocks, shallow or stopped breathing. Track the state of your jaw tension continuously. Try resting the tip of your tongue behind the front teeth or between the teeth. An open mouth is a sure sign of a relaxed jaw. Release happens in the presence of relaxation.

What do I need to know about yin yoga?

If you lead a typical life in this culture it is jam-packed with productivity and activity. When we choose recreation it often has the same qualities. When we decide we need to fit in yoga because we heard it was good for us, we choose active yang styles. Yin yoga is about quieting, turning inward, cultivating a peaceful receptivity. For many of us, it is the perfect balance to an active life style.

That being said, yin yoga is not for every body. If you were born naturally limber and can sit on the floor legs wide and flop your chest and belly on the floor, this may not be the best physical practice for you. You may enjoy it for the meditative aspects or for specific injuries that have resulted in connective tissue restriction. But creating increased laxity in an already gumby-like body does not make sense. For this population, a practice that focuses on stability and strength is sometimes more appropriate. It is a mistake to be drawn to any practice simply because it is easy for you.

For the rest of us stiff types, we must learn to patiently come into each yin pose and spend the first minute making all the physical adjustments needed to find our edge. Sometimes we use soft props like blankets, bolsters and pillows to support the weight of the body at our edge. Sinking further into the stretch as structures release is possible when the props are soft. We don't use effort to create more range of motion. We simply let gravity have her way with us. I love to do this practice in bed: the softness of the mattress, · the warmth of the blankets, the support of the pillows create a wonderful practice nest!

This is a yoga that is more about sensation than form. When we find our yin edge, the connective tissue between the bones has been stressed enough to soften. Sometimes the sensation is one of compression as structures press into each other. Sometimes the feeling is lengthening tension or traction as structures are being separated. Learn to feel the difference in these two distinct sensations.

After the first minute of adjustments, resolve to still the body and quiet the breath. Use this template of stillness as a guide to empty the mind. Hold this surrendered state for 2-5 minutes and focus on the sensation in the target area and the breath.

Come out of the pose slowly. Experiment with using the in-breath or the out-breath to ease out of the position. Take a few moments to create some gentle movement or come into an opposite direction pose (a counter pose) for a few moments. Focus on the post-pose sensation. If there is no lingering sensation you have yet to find a way to affect change in the target. There will often be a temporary feeling of fragility and vulnerability in the target area that may feel like heat, tingling or aching. This is a sign that the connective tissue has been stressed and the sensation should dissipate within a minute.

If discomfort lasts longer than a minute, it is important to note that you may have pushed beyond your edge. I am reminded of a new yoga student who repeatedly reported, "The yoga hurt me". There is so much to learn about bringing 100% of our attention to the moment and how to come right up to our edge without pushing or efforting beyond it. If you have had a "too much" experience, resolve to come in more gently, more slowly, more attentively in the next pose.

What if I have a problem with my nerves?

As we move, healthy nerve fibers move freely through the tissues of the body. When problems in the muscles, connective tissue and joints are chronic or if we undergo an acute and severe injury, the nervous system often becomes involved. Injuries often create areas of scarring that ensnare and tether the nerve fibers.

Pain, numbness or tingling that starts in the neck or low back and travels into the arm or leg can be radiating from a nerve. Any technique or pose that brings on or intensifies a symptom of this nature takes very special consideration. Often symptoms from the nervous system are irritated with prolonged pressure or stretching.

If this applies to you, know that when you come out of a pressure technique or pose, any symptom change you create should be gone within a minute. If the symptom change persists, you have been too aggressive and will need to explore a modification. Sometimes it can be pretty complicated finding a way that is best for you. This is definitely a sign to consider some professional expert help. In this guide, the angel wing test and breathing with pelvic motion are included as individual patient guides. Get to know your body by experimenting gently and carefully; consider supportive help from a physical therapist if you need it.

How important is strength?

In the presence of connective tissue tightness, muscular strength is always compromised. It is not only a waste of effort to do strengthening exercises in the presence of tightness, it can actually create or aggravate existing pain. Even though I am a physical therapist, it has been years since I have believed in exercising specifically for strength. As constricted areas unwind, the muscles that keep us in motion are in a more optimal position to come into their natural power and normal function.

As we release what is tight, a practice of functional core stability will put us in touch with our emerging natural power. Practicing this skill will help to maintain release. I have taught core stabilization for years in the physical therapy world. The ancient yogis had this one dialed in a long time ago. Bhanda is the yogic term for the locks that provide internal structural support for our alignment. Bhandas also have an energetic function: the movement of energy in the chakras from the base of the spine to the crown. In yin practice, bhanda power will increase or decrease the tension in some poses. It will also connect the core to the feet in standing poses and protect your spine out in the real world.

You can experiment with engaging the bhandas while sitting, standing or laying down. This is an awareness practice that will continue to grow over many, many years:

• *Root lock:* on the exhale, gently draw the lower belly toward back body and softly lift the pelvic floor into the body without clenching or gripping. "Gently" is the key word here.

• *Neck lock:* on the inhale, lengthen the back of the neck, like a kitten being lifted by a mother cat. Drop the chin slightly, softly lift the breastbone and melt the wingtips of the shoulder blades down the back body.

• *Diaphragm lock:* on the inhale, gently lift the heart center away from the belly; on the exhale draw the diaphragm muscle up and in.

Application of the bhandas will increase and decrease sensation in many of the poses. When we combine the breath with the bhandas they serve as an anchor for our attention in mindful meditation during the poses.

What about the breath?

There is no "right way" to breath when releasing with the balls and rollers or during the yin poses. The flow of breath just needs to keep continually coming. That being said, it is quite beautiful to make the release work a complete meditative yoga practice. That happens when we bring 100% of our attention into body sensation and breath at the same time we practice the techniques and poses.

There are many ways to pay attention to the breath. Choose one and stay with this focus throughout one complete session. Here are some starting ideas you can choose to focus on:

• Movement of breath in the belly

• Sensation of breath in the throat

• Pauses in the breath at the top of the inhale and/or the bottom of the exhale

• Counting breaths

• Timing the length of the breath, making inhale and exhale equal

How about incorporating mindful meditation in my practice?

Whether we practice meditation on its own or in the context of the release work, we will experience many positive benefits. Most regular meditators feel the gift of reduced anxiety and physical pain. Modern technology and the new field of contemplative neuroscience have studied how the brain changes with meditation. Brain scans of meditators show more connections between brain cells and increased networks of blood vessels. This is especially noticeable in areas that control our ability to focus attention, be self-aware and feel empathy. Reductions in pain and anxiety are correlated with physical changes in the amygdala, the brain structure that plays a role in anxiety and stress. Integrating mindful meditation into your release practice can bear some great fruit.

We apply the technique of mindful meditation with discipline AND gentle compassion. There are no whips or chains involved; there is no wrong way to do it. The most seasoned meditators have the same distractions. Here are the concrete and simple steps to mindful meditation:

- Anchor in the breath: choose a breath focus and continue to come back to it.

- Anchor in the target area: bring your attention to sensation in the target region. Experiment with directing the flow of breath to this area.

- Gently accept and label distractions as they arise. Distractions take us away from focusing on breath and sensation. They generally fall into two categories:

    Thoughts - name the thought as soon as you notice it arising: planning, reviewing, rehearsing, judging, anxiety. It's a long and endless list. It is what the brain is paid to do.

    Emotions - name the feeling as soon as you notice it arising: afraid, sad, happy, content, angry. Another long and endless list. It is what the heart does.

- Come back to the anchor. A thousand times we come back. Again and again we gently return to the breath, we come back to our focus on sensation.

How do I combine breath and bhandas?

Keeping the attention on the breath without incorporating the bhandas is a perfect practice with the rollers and the balls. If you are new to the yin poses, attention on the breath alone is enough. There are so many elements at play as we learn to combine breath and bhandas. It can take many years to weave this tapestry of awareness. Take your time slowly integrating whatever pieces you actually feel. Try following one simple thread at a time before combining elements.

Since root lock is most easily felt during the out breath and neck lock is easiest to access on the in breath, we can learn to use this merge as our meditation anchor in many of the yin poses.

On the exhale: apply root lock to gently draw in the pelvic floor and deep abdominals. In many of the poses this creates an increased sensation of lengthening tension in the front of the hips, decreased sensation of compression in the low back and stabilization of the lumbar spine.

On the inhale: apply neck lock to draw the chin slightly down and open the back of the neck. This will also expand the rib cage, lift the breast bone and draw the shoulder blades down the back body. In many of the poses this creates a sense of length to the full spine. The inhale relaxes the pelvic floor open and often increases the sensation of compression in the spine.

Here are four ways to utilize the breath and bhanda marriage as your meditation. Read the specific instructions given with each pose and incorporate these techniques when you are ready. Experiment and discover which visualization rings true for you.

• *Crown to Root Breath:* We know that the breath actually enters the body through the mouth or nose but imagine the inhale entering an opening in the top of the head, the crown. Feel it enter the body and create neck lock. Lengthen the back of the neck, drop the chin and lift the breastbone. Exhale and follow the breath down the body creating the root lock. Draw the deep abdominals toward the back, close the pelvic floor and send roots into the earth.

• *Circle Breath:* Imagine the inhale originating at the tailbone. Follow it up the lengthening spine. Let it slowly create neck lock as it rounds the crown and lands at the point between the eyebrows at the top of the inhale. Feel the fullness of the neck lock in this moment. Exhale and follow the breath down the body. Create the root lock by drawing the deep abdominals toward the back and closing the pelvic floor.

· *Integrating Breath:* Imagine the inhale coming in through the heart and dropping to the pelvic floor. Let it create the neck lock and relax open the floor of the pelvis. Start the exhale by closing the pelvic floor and creating the root lock. Imagine this action and the corresponding drawing in of the deep abdominals as the energetic push of the breath back up to the heart.

• *Egg Breath:* Imagine the entire core from the top ribs and collar bones to the floor of the pelvis as a soft and expandable egg. Let the in breath, with the help of neck lock, open the rib cage, expand the trunk and push open the floor of the pelvis. Let the out breath, with the help of root lock, shrink the whole egg: the ribs descending, the deep belly drawing in, the floor of the pelvis drawing up.

Ready to roll

These opening paragraphs introduce the basic elements of an active release practice. The practical information that follows will guide you in creative exploration of your own body. Take time to slowly progress through this section. Allow the logic of the approach to shape your journey. Choose a target area to explore and begin by identifying and releasing the tightness with the roller, balls or your hands. Be curious about differences between the right and the left side. Next, surrender into the accompanying yin pose and give the connective tissue an opportunity to lengthen. Stay mindful by focusing the attention on sensation, breath and bhandas.

Many explorers want to go right to the areas of pain. We forget that tightness in seemingly unrelated areas often create the symptoms. Systematically assess your entire body with patience, love and an open curiosity. Most especially, relax and enjoy the ride. This is your unique and precious body. Give it some consistent attention over a period of time and you will be amazed at the way it responds and changes. It is just waiting for some of your love!

target: upper back

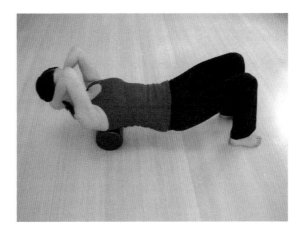

release: foam roller, upper back

Support your head so that front neck muscles stay totally relaxed. Lift hips or leave them in contact with the floor. Keep the chin tucked in as the elbows approach each other. Slowly roll from the "hump" at the base of your neck to the bottom of the shoulder blades. Pause at different locations. Focus on the out breath to let go.

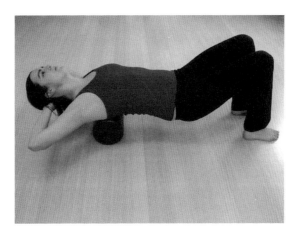

When closed elbows is easy, lean back into your hands, release the chin from the chest and open your elbows. Keep the body parallel to the floor. Gentle root lock keeps the low back from over arching and will focus the release in the upper back. This is an opportunity to un-hunch an area that spends so much time caved forward. Keep focused on the exhale for release.

release: tennis balls, upper back

Place the double balls perpendicular to the spine just below the "hump" at the base of neck. If your chin points up, use a enough pillow under the head so the face is parallel to the floor. Beyond your edge? Add an extra blanket, rug or mat. Cradle the shoulders with the hands and rock side to side to release tightness often felt on one side more than the other. Exhale to release, visualizing the back rib cage melting toward the floor. Come back to the center and lift hips to "scoot" to the next level down. Repeat the rocking, breathing, and scooting until you reach the bottom of the shoulder blades.

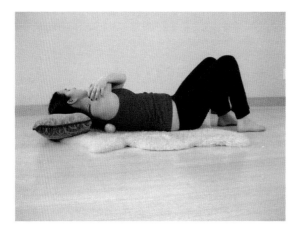

Ready for more edge? Come to a harder surface, remove the pillow support and move your extended arms side to side, overhead or asymmetrically. Move the arms in any fashion that feels releasing to the mid-back. Keep the breath coming continuously. Exhale to release and visualize the back rib cage melting toward the floor. Lift hips to "scoot" to the next level down and repeat breathing and arm motion until you reach the bottom of the shoulder blades. Keep the chin tucked and the low back flat to focus the pressure on the upper back.

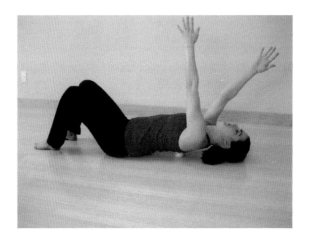

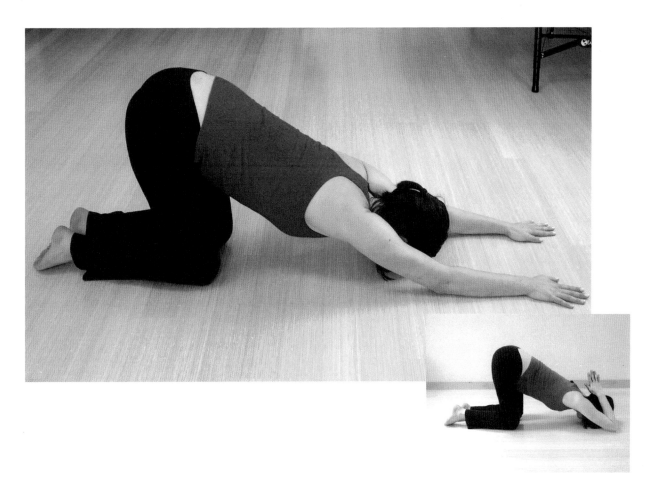

pose: puppy

Position the knees directly under the hips, extending both arms forward. Let the forehead rest on the floor, propping it on a soft blanket if needed. Allow the heart center to melt toward the floor and focus on the upper back target area. Feel the gentle ski slope of the entire spine. To increase the physical sensation in the shoulders, bend the elbows and bring namaste hands to the base of the neck. Apply neck lock to lengthen the spine and root lock to traction open the low back and deepen into the fold.

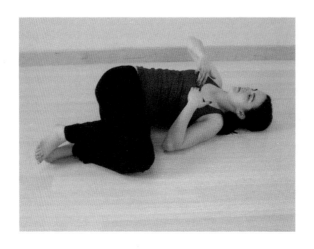

release: front rib

The tightness in front of the rib cage matches the tightness in the upper back. Lay on your left side and rotate open to the right. Use your fingers or base of palm to massage open the right chest, helping the shoulder to ease toward the floor. Focus on gently pulling each rib away from the breast bone and separating the ribs from each other. Find those particularly tight or tender areas and exhale to release. If you are using tennis balls to release thoracic spine, you can try this technique concurrently. This is also a great technique to apply in saddle pose and all the laying twists.

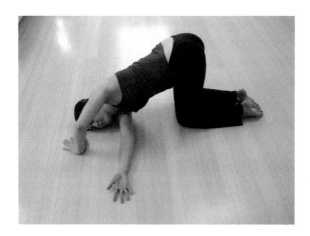

pose: twist, hand & knee

Position the knees directly under the hips. Reach the right arm through the space between the left knee and left arm, resting the right shoulder or shoulder blade on the floor. Let the left hand press into the floor to adjust into the edge of the twist. The left hand can stay on the floor or rest behind the back. Feel the upper back and rib cage opening into the turn. Apply neck lock to lengthen the rotated spine and root lock to deepen into the twist.

target: lower back

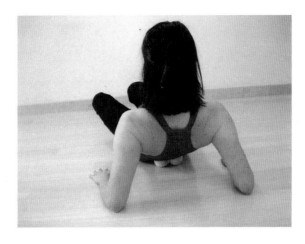

release: tennis balls, low back to sacrum

Place the balls across the spine, an inch or two below the shoulder blades. Pressure over your edge? Lift the hips enough to create the edge you need. You can also prop on the elbows to ease some of the pressure or use an extra blanket, rug or mat. Gently rock the knees back and forth and work the tightness you may feel on one side more than the other. Use the exhale to release. Lift hips to "scoot" to the next level down and repeat breathing, leg motion and scooting until you reach the sacrum.

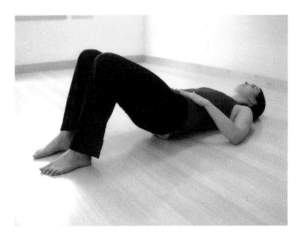

Place balls under sacrum and move knees back and forth or draw knees into the chest. You can also turn the balls 90 degrees and massage the sacrum from side to side.

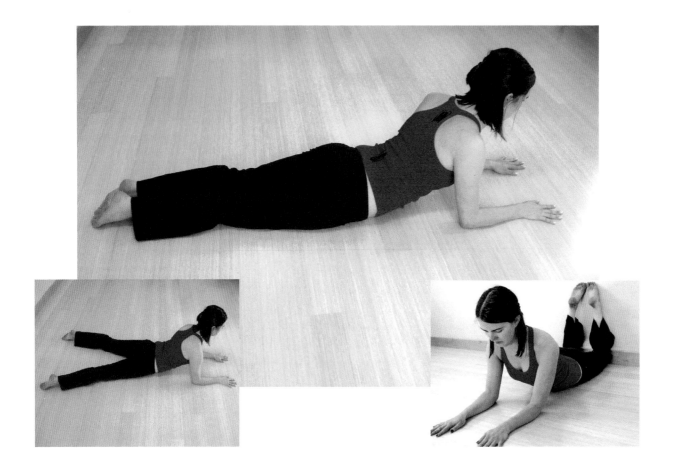

pose: sphinx

Place the elbows directly under the shoulders, forearms flat on the floor, palms down. Relax the buttocks. Focus on the sensation of compression in the low back and find your edge with these variations:

- Legs together or legs apart

- Shoulders slumping toward ears or actively drawing the shoulders down and back

- Elbows under the shoulders or positioned more in front of shoulders

- For deepening: a folded blanket under the forearms or legs up the wall.

Apply neck lock to lengthen the spine and deepen the sensation of compression. Apply root lock to momentarily stabilize the low back and decrease the sensation of compression.

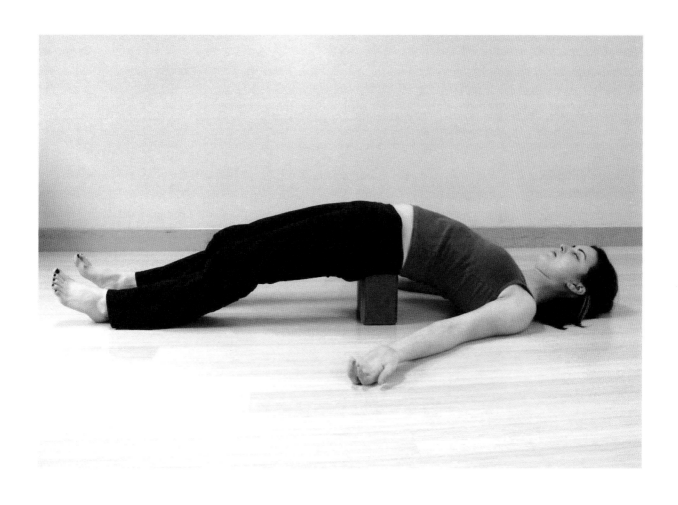

pose: supported bridge, legs extended

Use a yoga block under the sacrum to find your edge in the low, medium or high position. Slowly extend legs and feel for compression in the low back and lengthening tension in front of the hips.

Apply neck lock to lengthen the spine and root lock to stabilize and momentarily decompress the low back and increase sensation in front of the hips.

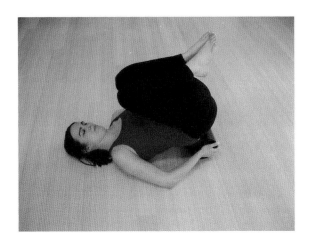

release: foam roller, child's pose

Lift hips in a bridge and place the roller underneath the sacrum. Hold the sides of the roller and allow the knees to descend toward the chest. Focus on the opening sensation of lengthening tension in the lower back. Shift the roller higher or lower to target where it is most needed in your low back. Breathe continuously. Applying root lock on the exhale will increase sensation.

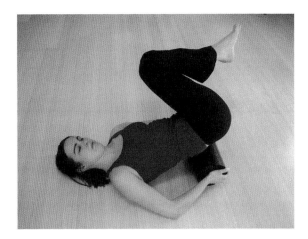

Experiment with the massage that happens rocking the knees from side to side. Find a way to marry the breath with this motion.

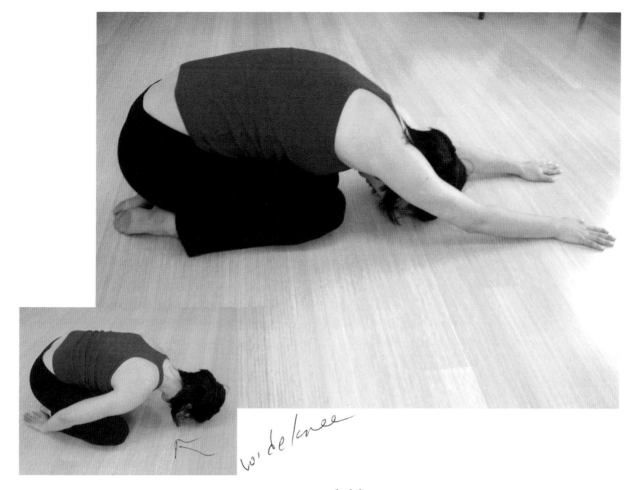

wide knee

pose: child

From hands and knees, let the hips descend toward the heels. If the forehead does not touch the ground, use a soft blanket under it. Too edgy for the knees? Place a blanket between the calf and the back of the thigh. Focus on the sensation of lengthening tension in the low back and find your edge with these variations:

· Knees close together or wide apart

· Arms extended forward, palms down

· Arms forward, palms stacked with forehead resting on back of hands

· Arms back, palms up next to soles of feet

Apply neck lock to lengthen the spine. Apply root lock to traction open the low back and deepen into the fold.

target: neck & shoulder

The base of the skull often has very specific tight spots that can be the source of headache pain. Release the area at the base of the head with these two techniques, exhaling to release each tight spot.

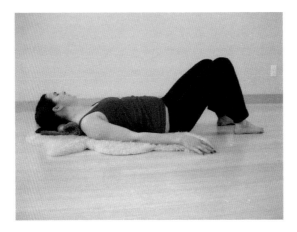

release: tennis balls, head

Use a small rolled hand towel in the curve of the neck and place the tennis balls just above. Massage this region by rolling the head right and left, like the gesture of "no". When you find a tight spot, pause and move the head up and down in the gesture of "yes".

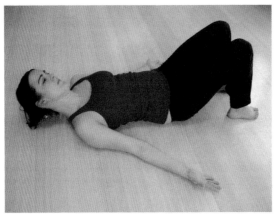

release: pokey ball, head

Place the pokey ball along the skull ridge and use no and yes movements to release this target area.

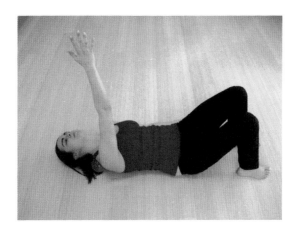

release: shoulder blade balls

Place ball at the upper corner of shoulder blade. Exhale to release any tightness. Keep your head relaxed on the ground and shift your hips so the ball travels to all the places on the shoulder blade border. Breathe and release at each tight spot. Add movements of the arm on the same side for more pressure. Too edgey? Support your head with a pillow and/or roll toward the opposite side for less pressure.

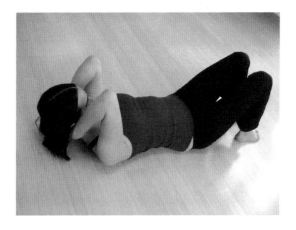

pose: head cradle

Support the weight of the head with clasped hands. Let the index fingers be parallel to the skull line. Let the thumbs angle down the back of the neck. Ask the front neck muscles to completely let go of all effort and gently guide the chin toward the chest. Continue to let gravity do the job of drawing the back of the neck toward the floor. Feel the sensation of lengthening tension develop in the target area behind the neck. Keep the jaw relaxed. Apply neck lock to lengthen the spine and relax open the pelvic floor.

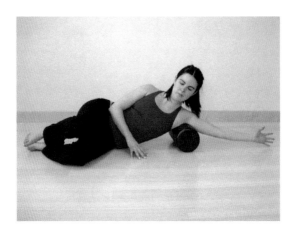

release: foam roller, under arm

Lay on left side, knees and hips flexed up. Place roller under upper arm. Roll the tender area from just above the armpit to the upper rib cage. Pause to breathe and release any particularly tight spots.

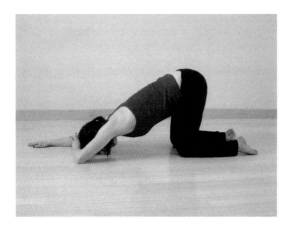

pose: puppy, one arm

Position the knees directly under the hips, extending the right arm forward. Place the left palm in the crease of the right elbow. Allow the forehead to rest on the left forearm. Feel the heart center melt toward the floor and focus on letting go in the target area throughout the right shoulder and mid back.

Apply gentle neck lock to lengthen the spine and secure the neutral placement of the head. Apply root lock to stabilize the low back.

target: shoulder, elbow, wrist

The next four poses focus on the connective tissue around the shoulder, elbow and wrist. Establish the neck lock and feel the full length of the spine. Apply root lock to counteract the tendency to over arch the low back in these poses.

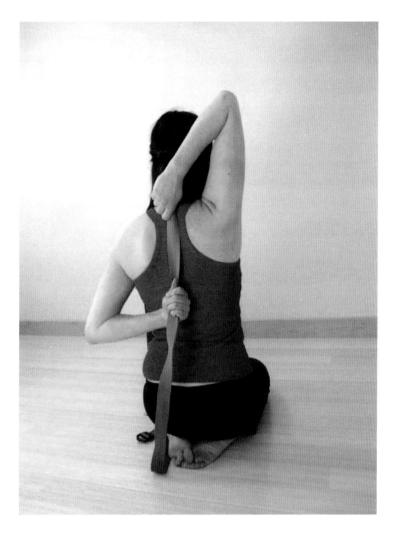

pose: behind the back reach

Sit with neutral alignment. Reach right arm up, shoulder externally rotated, palm turned inward. Bend elbow, letting palm approach shoulder blades. Reach left arm down, shoulder internally rotated. Bend elbow, left palm turned outward and approach shoulder blades from below. Clasp hands together or hold a strap to maintain the release. Feel the sensation of lengthening tension differently in both triceps and shoulders.

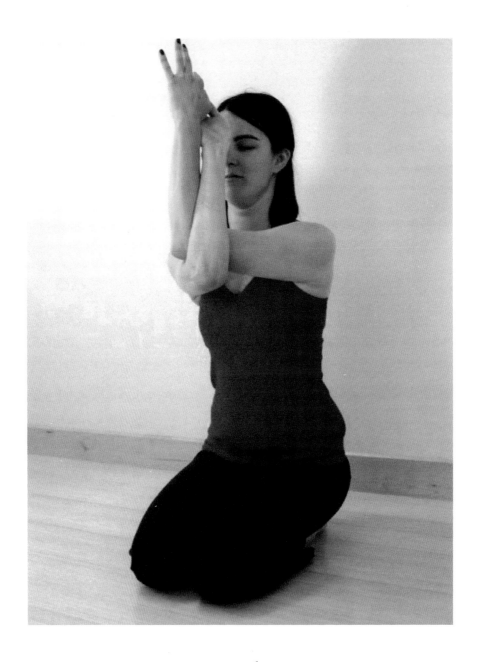

pose: eagle arms

Sit with neutral alignment. Reach across body with left arm on top, giving yourself a hug by holding as much of the shoulder blade as possible. Stay right here if this is your edge of lengthening tension in between the shoulder blades. If you are able to rotate the shoulders and bring the back of the hands or the palms together, add this variation. Lift the lower arm so it is parallel to the floor and draw the elbow points away from the body. You can rest into the pose more deeply by bending forward at the hips and resting the right elbow on the floor.

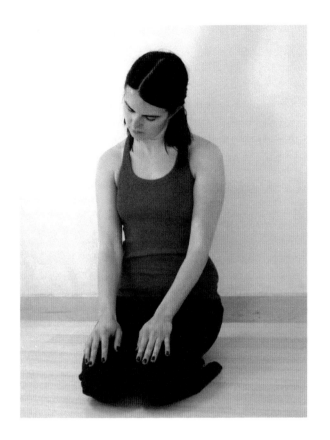 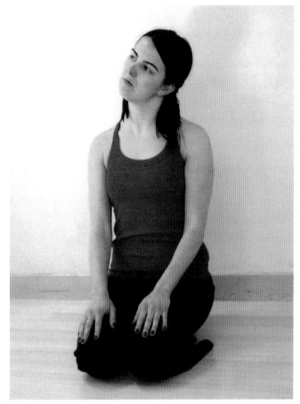

pose: neck, 2 way

Sit with neutral alignment and keep right shoulder blade down and back. Side bend the left ear toward the left shoulder . Stay right here if this is your edge of lengthening tension on the right side of the neck. To increase the sensation down toward the right shoulder blade, look down toward the left armpit. To increase sensation toward the right side of the head, look up and to the right just a little.

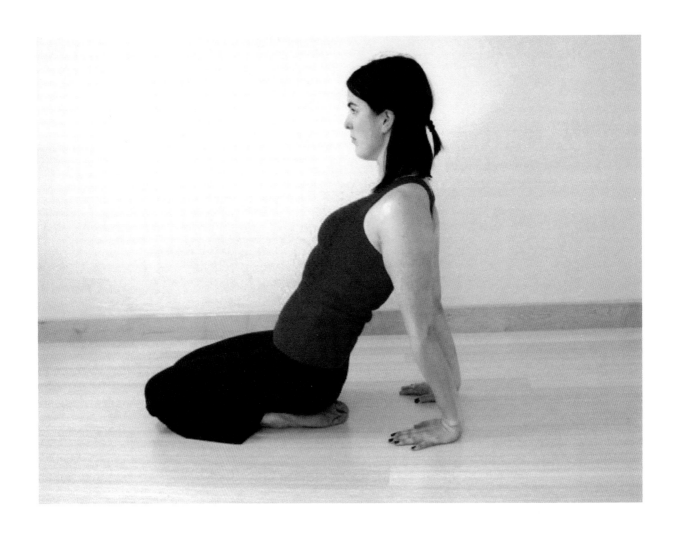

pose: wrist opener

Start by sitting in neutral alignment. Internally rotate both shoulders, lift the heart center and place the palms as flat as possible on the floor. Feel the sensation of lengthening tension throughout the wrist and the palm side of the forearm.

target: full spine

release: tennis balls, full spine

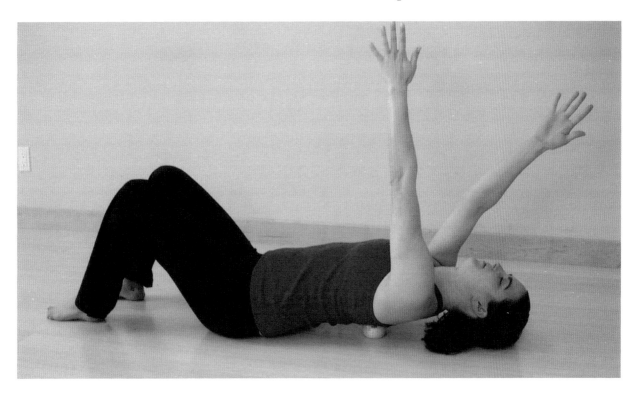

Take the tennis ball journey from the base of the neck, exploring all the way down to the sacrum. Breathe and release at each distinct level. Use movements of the arms and legs to focus the pressure more on one side than the other. Track and release any holding or tension in other regions especially around the face, the jaw, the buttocks. Discover and love your spine!

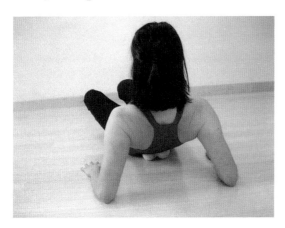

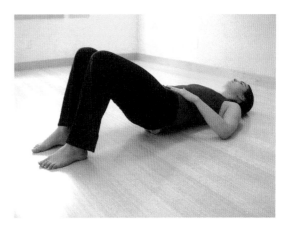

pose: twist, full spine

Four ways to explore:

In all the twists you can apply gentle neck lock to lengthen the rotated spine and open the chest on the up side. Applying root lock will deepen you into the twist.

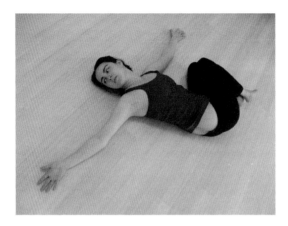

First try a twist in flexion: Lay on your left side, knees flexed deeply into chest. Rotate and open to the right, trying different arm positions to explore your edge on the right chest, low back, hip and side of the leg. Repeat on the other side.

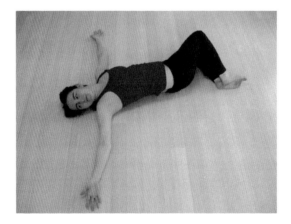

Feel the difference when you twist in extension: Lay on your left side with hips flexed to less than a right angle, knees flexed. Rotate and open to the right, trying different arm positions to explore your edge on the right chest, low back, hip and side of the leg. Repeat other side.

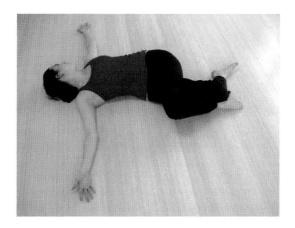

For a very different sensation, twist, cross knees: Lay on back and cross left knee over right. Spread the arms wide. Allow the weight of legs to fall to the right and look left. Try different arm positions to explore your edge on the left chest, low back, hip and side of the leg. Repeat on other side.

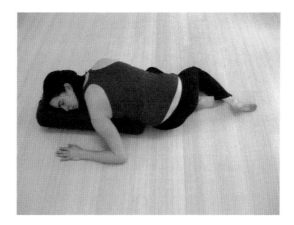

For a soft, supported feel, twist, prone: Side sit on the left hip, knees folded under. Turn the belly and chest completely to the left and then descend to the floor. Prop on a bolster or pillow if needed. Experiment with turning the head to the left if possible. Too edgey for the neck? Keep it turned to the right. Repeat on other side.

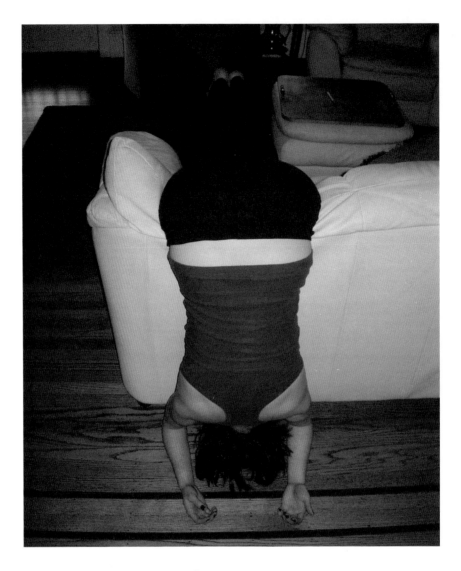

release: traction

Sometimes it is useful to keep the entire spine fairly neutral and apply a separating traction to all the connective tissue holding the vertebral column. Depending on your actual length and weight, there is often furniture at home that will support this. Check out this picture of hanging over the top of a couch to get you thinking. Supported at the hip crease and top of the thighs, knees bent, there is full surrender of the weight of the trunk. For safety, have someone close by to assist the first time. While they are at it, what a great opportunity to receive a massage all through the hips and back!

Apply gentle neck lock to lengthen the tractioned spine. On the exhale, lightly draw up and in on the pelvic floor and deep abdominals to traction open the low back more fully.

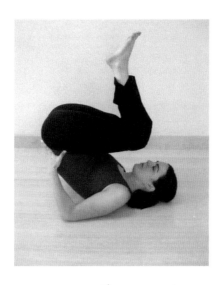

pose: snail progression

This is an advanced pose and benefits from release preparation in the spine and especially the neck before proceeding. When you are warmed up, place bent elbows on either side of the body, palms facing in. Draw the shoulder blades down the back by pressing the upper arm into the floor. Use the power of the deep abdominals to lift the hips. Support the back with the palms. Feel the sensation of lengthening tension throughout the entire neck and spine.

Apply neck lock to draw in the chin and lengthen the spine. Apply root lock to traction open the low back and deepen into the fold.

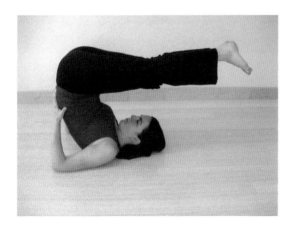
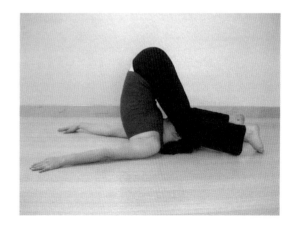

When you are ready to curl the spine more, try extending the legs, possibly touching the toes down to the floor or a perfectly placed bolster. Or let the knees bend and rest toward the ears.

pose: forward fold, standing

In all forward folds you can apply neck lock to lengthen the spine and apply root lock to open the lower back and deepen into the fold.

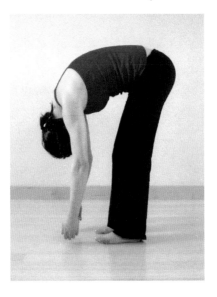

1. Stand with feet hip width apart, outer borders of the feet parallel to each other, knees softly unlocked. Release the chin to the chest, round the shoulders and fold forward. Feel the window of the low back open and the lengthening tension in the upper back. Feel the complete weight of the head dangling, a source of traction to the neck.

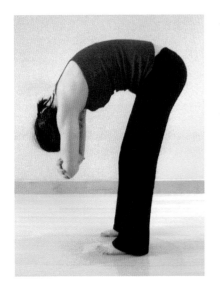

2. Position as in #1 and cup the elbows in the opposite hands.

3. Position as in #1 and back up to a wall so that the upper back is supported and the low back is gently coaxed into more of a fold.

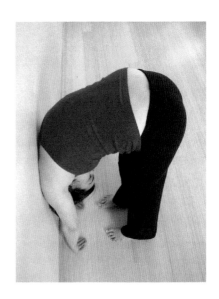

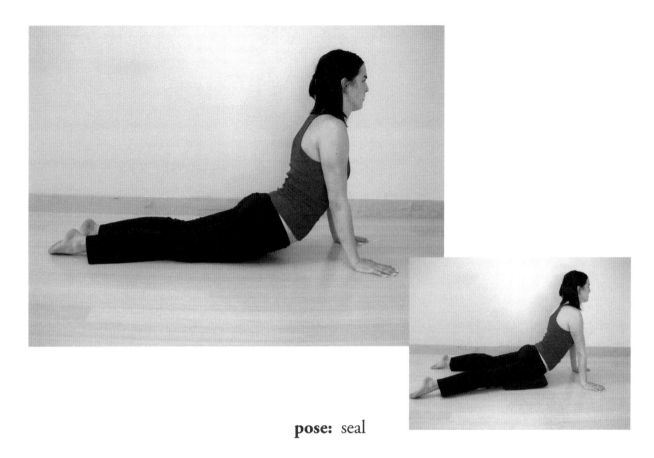

pose: seal

Lay on belly with palms under shoulders, hands turned out slightly. Press up until the elbows are straight. Focus on the compression sensation in the low back and possibly the upper back. Feel the lengthening tension in front of the hips and belly. Apply neck lock to lengthen the spine and deepen the sensation of compression. Apply root lock to momentarily stabilize the low back and decrease the sensation of compression.

Find your edge with these variations:

- Legs together or legs apart

- Shoulders slumping toward ears or actively drawing the shoulders down and back

- Hands under the shoulders or positioned more in front of shoulders

- A folded blanket under the pelvis to decrease sensation.

target: hips

release: roller, side leg

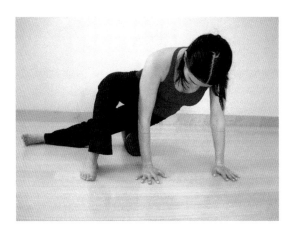

Lay on the roller about six inches down from the top of the hip. Create a tripod with both arms and the top leg. Take as much weight on the hands and the front supporting foot as needed to create the edge you need. Slowly massage the side region of the leg from the hip to the knee. Lean forward enough to also massage the area between the side and the front of the leg. Keep deep abdominals active and pause at extra tight sections to breathe and release. Avoid the bony area just above the knee and at the side of the hip bone. Initially this release can be quite painful. It is gratifying to witness our ability to change this connective tissue restriction. Regular attention will normalize the tissue. A healthy leg does not hurt when it is rolled.

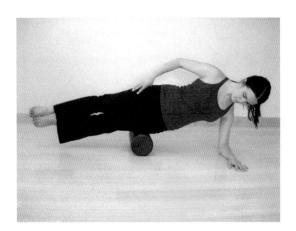

When you have really slowed down and found all the patches of tightness and the tripod method is too easy to be edgy, stack the legs and come down on elbow.

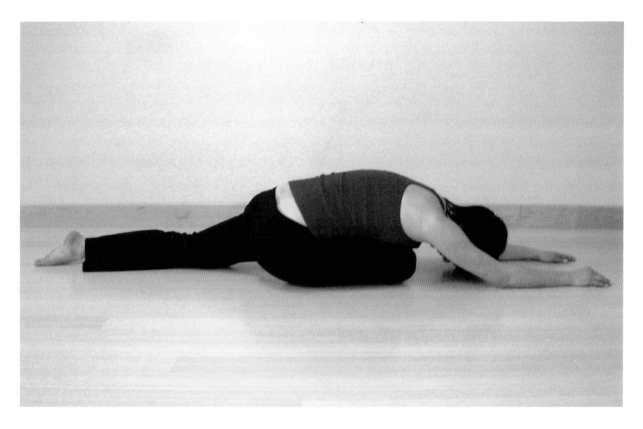

pose: swan, sleeping

Start on hands and knees. Draw the right knee up until the knee is between the wrists and shin is resting on the mat. Allow the upper body to sink down so the breast bone approaches or rests on the thigh. The right foot can rest in the groin or move toward the left armpit. Wiggle the hips back and forth searching for the position that creates lengthening tension in the side of the leg and/or deep in the right hip.

Decrease the target sensation by staying on the elbows or place a pillow or blanket under the right hip for support. Increase sensation by sinking the breast bone all the way to the leg. There will also be a more mild sensation at the front of the left hip. Extend the left leg further back to increase that sensation. Apply neck lock to lengthen the spine. Apply root lock to traction open the low back, deepen into the fold and increase sensation in front of the extended leg.

release: pokey ball, hip front

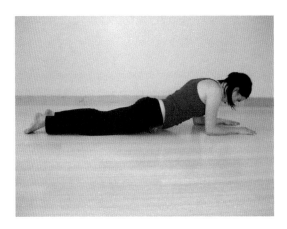

Prop on the elbows and place the ball in the "cup" at the front of the hip, level with the bone that juts out from the front of the pelvis. Try to catch the edge of the tissue as it comes off the inside front of the pelvic bone. Explore an inch or two up and down from this central starting point, exhaling at each tight spot for release.

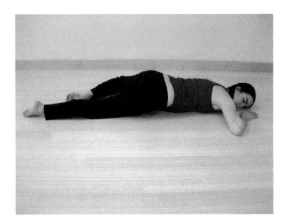

To increase the intensity of the pressure, allow the upper body to rest on the floor and/or bend the opposite hip and knee up along the floor. Keep breathing. Each exhale is an opportunity to let go.

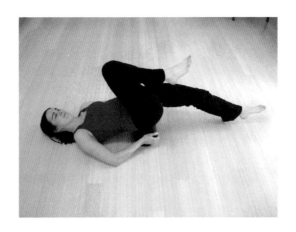

release: foam roller, hip front

Bridge up at the hips and slide the roller under the sacrum. Draw the right knee toward the chest. Extend the left leg toward the floor. Experiment with the roller position to search for just the right amount of right hip and knee bend and just the right amount of left leg extension. You can clasp your hands around the knee moving toward the chest. The front of the left hip is the target; find an edge of lengthening tension in this area. Apply gentle root lock on the exhale to intensify the sensation.

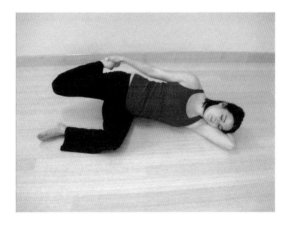

pose: leg pull

Lay on the left side. Bend both knees and hips as deeply as possible. Use the right hand to catch the right ankle, pulling the knee back so it is even with the body. Pull the heel toward the right hip. Feel the sensation of lengthening tension in front of the right thigh. Increase the sensation of compression in the low back, allowing it to arch by extending the bottom leg back along the floor. Try not to let the right knee drift upward.

Apply neck lock to lengthen the spine and open the rib cage. This will increase compression sensation in the low back. Apply root lock to stabilize and decrease sensation in the low back. This will increase sensation in the front of the thigh.

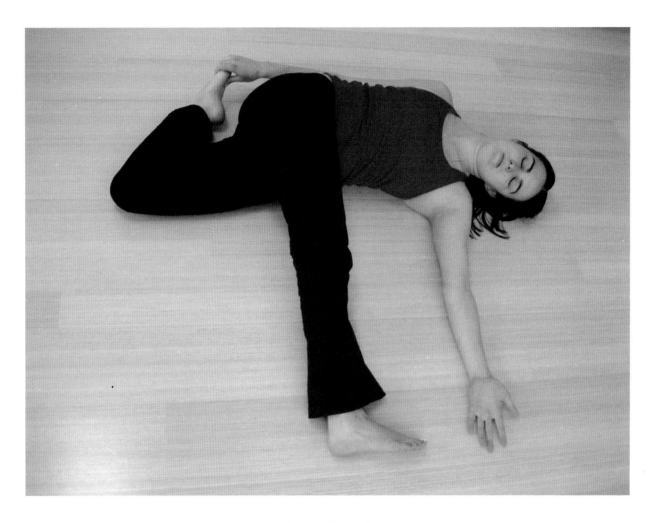

pose: leg pull with twist

Lay on the back, both legs straight. Extend the right leg to the ceiling. Keep the knee extended and the hip at a right angle; allow the leg to drop all the way to the left. "Scooch" the bottom left leg along the floor as far back as possible. Bend the left knee and use the right hand to catch the left foot, pulling the heel toward the left hip. Feel the sensation of lengthening tension in front of the left thigh and in the right low back and hip. Deepen the sensation by allowing the right upper body to open into a twist to the right.

Apply gentle neck lock to lengthen the spine and open the front of the upside rib cage. Apply root lock to draw more deeply into the twist. This will increase sensation in the front of the bottom thigh.

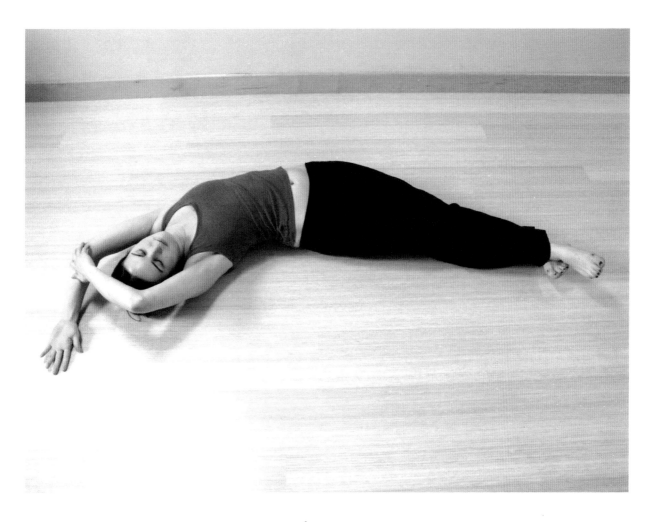

pose: banana asana

From a relaxed back laying pose, walk the legs to the right until there is a lengthening sensation on the outside of the left leg. Turn the left leg in and anchor it in place with the right ankle. Keep the left hip on the floor. Slowly walk the upper body to the right. Rest here or create more sensation in the left side rib cage by extending the cradled arms overhead.

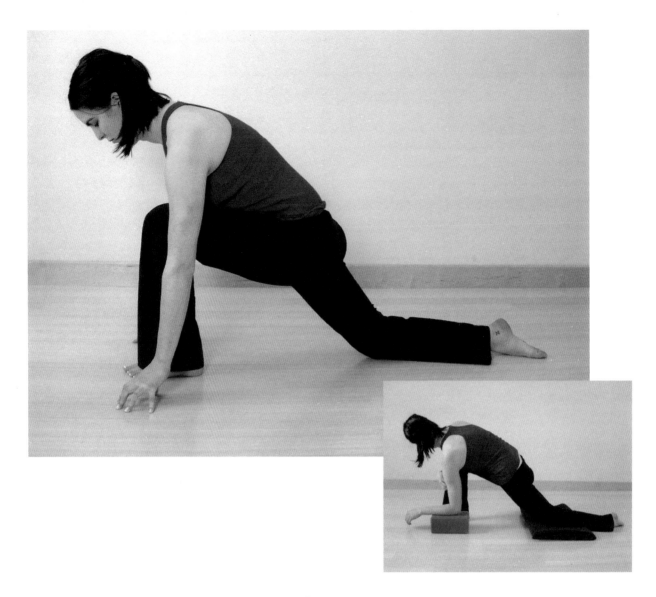

pose: lunge, resting

Come into a lunge position with the left knee over the ankle, hands resting on the floor on either side of the left foot. Allow the belly and/or chest to rest on the top of the left thigh. Scoot the right leg back until you feel the sensation of lengthening tension in front of the right hip. You can add on by hugging the front knee with the arm on the same side and dropping the other forearm to the floor or a block. Gently adding a twist away from the leg that is stretched back will intensify sensation in front of that hip.

Apply neck lock to lengthen the full spine. Apply root lock to stabilize the low back and increase sensation in front hip of the leg that is extended back.

pose: knee opener

This series of three progressive poses creates an internal lengthening sensation of the knee and you will need a ½ " (easier) to 1" (more aggressive) wooden dowel and 2 yoga blocks (or something of comparable height). Go very slowly with big respect for your edge and seek professional guidance if you have knee issues and feel unsure of the value of taking this on. Keep the heart lifted as much as possible and rest and breathe for one minute in each position. Notice how regular practice paves the way to less sensation. Adjust height of blocks and dowel size as you progress.

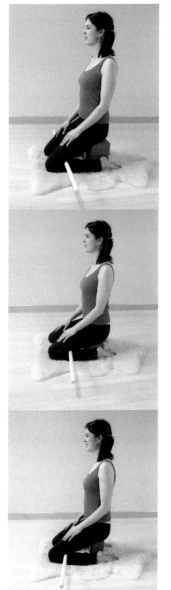

From kneeling, place dowel deep in the knee crease and sit back on 2 yoga blocks.

From kneeling, move the dowel back about 2-3 inches down the calf away from the knee crease. Sit back on one yoga block.

From kneeling, move the dowel back to the original position and sit back on one yoga block.

pose: frog high and low

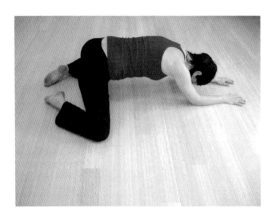

Come onto hands and knees with the hips positioned directly over the knees. Maintain this orientation as you allow the knees to slide apart. Feel for the sensation of lengthening tension along the inner thigh and groin.

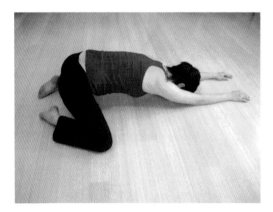

Experiment with letting the hips move back toward the heels and choose the position that creates the best edge of sensation in the inner thigh for you.

Apply neck lock to feel the full available relaxation of the pelvic floor and lengthen the spine. Apply root lock to deepen sensation in the inner thighs.

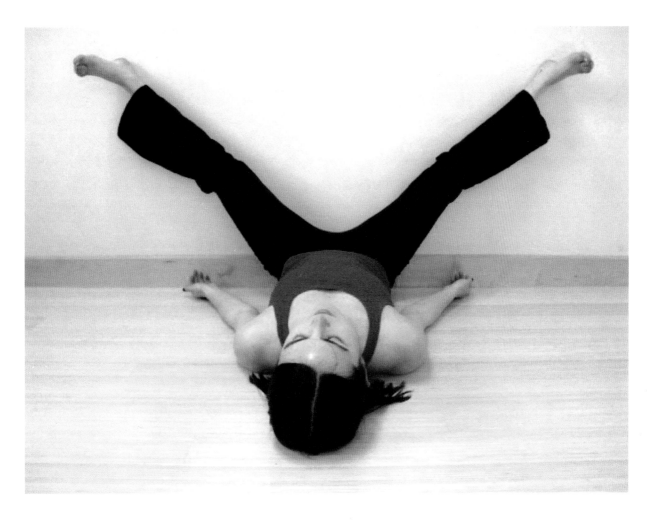

pose: legs up wall

Scoot hips right up to the wall and begin the pose with legs together. Slowly release legs open, coming to your edge gradually. Feel the lengthening tension in the inner thigh, possibly all the way to the inner knee.

Apply neck lock to relax the pelvic floor open and feel the full length of the spine supported by the floor. Apply root lock to feel support for the low back.

target: hip & low back

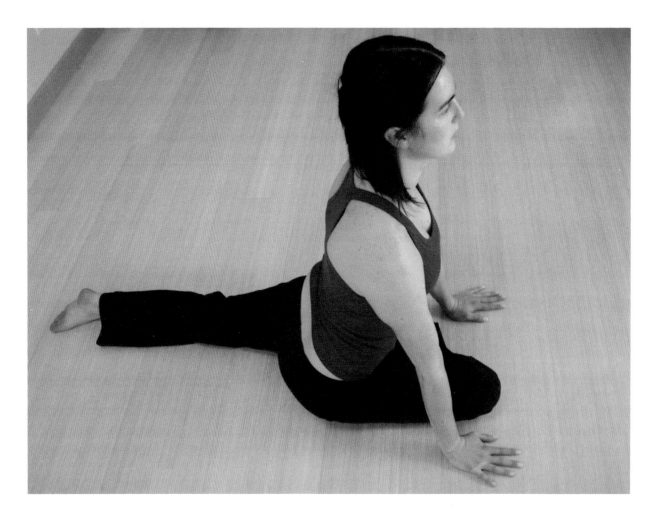

pose: swan, awake

From hands and knees draw the right knee up between the wrists resting the shin on the mat. The right foot can rest in the groin or begin to approach the left hand. Press into the hands and extend the low back enough to feel compression. Increase the tension at the front of the left hip by extending the left leg further back. Wiggle the hips back and forth to find the edge of sensation in the right side leg and/or deep in the right hip.

In this pose and the lunge that follows apply neck lock to drop the chin, lengthen the spine and deepen into the backbend. Apply root lock to stabilize and decompress the low back and increase sensation in front of the hip on the extended leg.

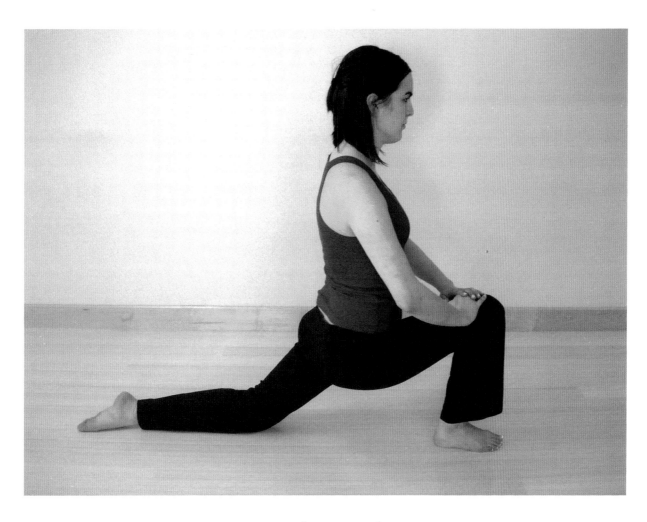

pose: lunge, awake

Come into a lunge position with the right knee directly over the ankle, hands resting on the floor on either side of the right foot. Scoot the left leg back until you feel the sensation of lengthening tension in front of the left hip. Place the hands on the right thigh and bring the upper body perpendicular to the floor, creating the sensation of compression on the low back.

Once you are comfortable with sphinx or seal and lunge experiment with saddle pose variations. The sensation of lengthening tension will be in the front body: the thigh, hip, and under the bottom of the rib cage. There will also be compression sensation in the low back.

You can ease into the pose by simply coming to the hands or elbows first and maintaining the posture right here. Come out carefully and breathing continuously. Some people lift the knees and come out. Many roll to one side slowly and release. Some find it helpful to push into the feet with the hands, tractioning open the spine and then lifting to the elbows first.

Apply neck lock to lengthen the spine and open the rib cage. This will increase compression sensation in the low back. Apply root lock to stabilize and decrease sensation in the low·back. This will increase sensation in the front of the thigh.

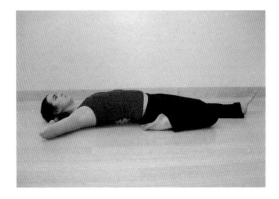

half saddle: From sitting, bend the left hip and knee and fold the leg under. Rest back on hands or elbows. Lay back on the floor for a deeper edge.

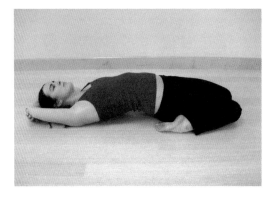

full saddle: From sitting on knees, lean back on hands or elbows and stay right here if this creates your edge. Lay back on the floor for a deeper edge.

To ease the sensation of saddle:

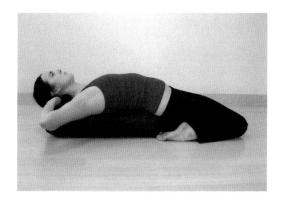

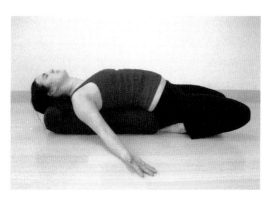

- Stay up on hands or elbows or prop a bolster, pillows or blankets from the low back to the head

- Allow the knees to be wide and/or lifted off the floor

- Keep the arms by your side

- Sit on the heels

To increase the sensation of saddle:

- Decrease or eliminate the propping from low back to head

- Draw the knees closer together and/or rest them on the floor

- Bring the arms overhead

- Sit between the heels

- Use your hands to massage open the ribs, explore the connection of the diaphragm under the rib cage or delve into the front of the pelvis

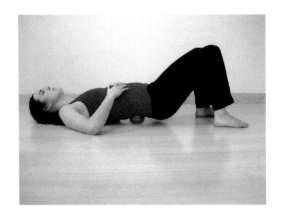

release: pokey ball, waist

Lift your hips and place the ball along your waistline, above the upper edge of your pelvic bone. Lower and shift your hips so the ball moves back and forth along the edge of your pelvis. "Dig out" this valley and find the tightest spots to breathe into and release. Sometimes they are so far over you need to almost roll onto your side.

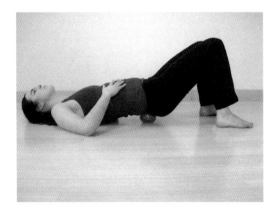

release: pokey ball, hip back

Lift your hips and place the ball under your buttocks, just below the edge of the pelvis. Explore the upper part of your hip, pausing to breathe and release tight spots. Try straightening and bending the leg on that side or even drawing the knee into the chest. Find what creates pressure in the target area most effectively.

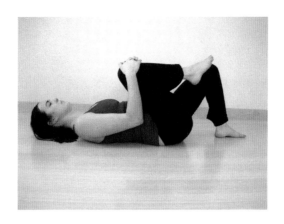

pose: knee to chest, single

Draw one knee to chest and feel for the sensation of lengthening tension created at the waist and in the back of the hip. Create more of an edge by extending the opposite leg onto the floor.

With both single and double knee to chest, relax the pelvic floor open and apply neck lock to lengthen the spine. Apply root lock to open the low back and deepen into the fold.

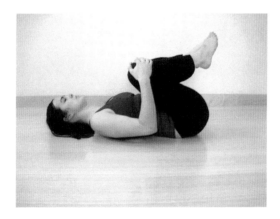

pose: knee to chest, double

Draw both knees together and pull them toward the chest. Feel for the sensation of lengthening tension created at the waist and in the back of both hips. Feel the difference when the knees are wide. Choose the position that creates the sensation edge just right for you.

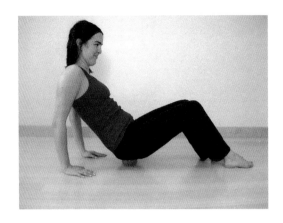

release: pokey ball, hip sit

Sit resting back on hands. Place the ball just above (and a little to the outside of) the sit bone and explore for tightness, pausing to breathe and release. Try straightening and bending the leg on that side at different angles to find what creates the most effective release.

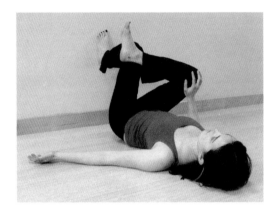

pose: figure 4

Lay on back a few inches from the wall, knees and hips bent, feet on wall. Extend the right leg to the ceiling and turn the knee and foot out. Bend the knee and place the outside of the right ankle on the left thigh. Draw the toes toward the knees and push the right knee away from you. Feel for the sensation of lengthening tension deep in the posterior right hip. Create more edge by drawing the left knee toward the chest or scooting the hips closer to the wall. Keep the weight balanced equally on the sacrum.

Apply neck lock to lengthen the spine and drop the chin. Apply root lock to deepen sensation in the hip.

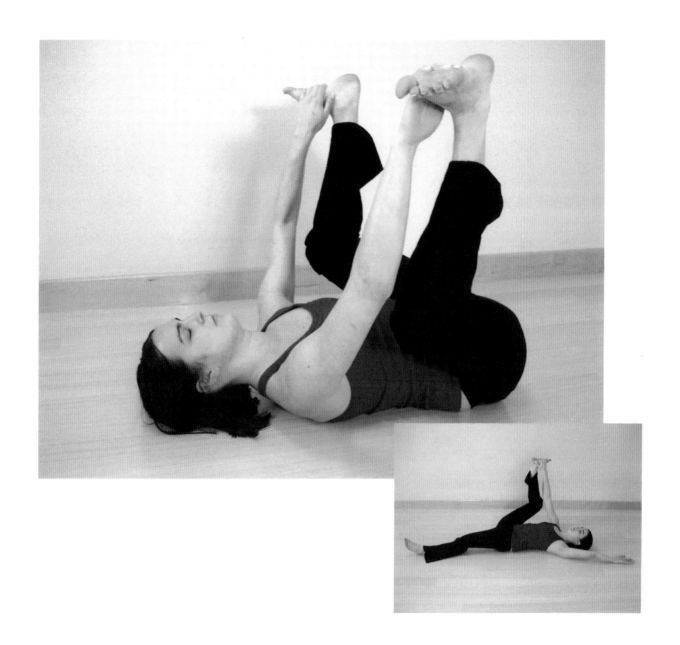

pose: happy baby

Draw the knees toward the armpits. With the arms inside the knees, hold the feet on the inside or outside arch and deepen into the sensation of lengthening tension in the posterior hip and anterior groin. If the feet are not reachable, hold the shins or behind the knees. Release one leg and tune in to the lengthening sensation in front of the extended hip.

Apply neck lock to lengthen the spine and relax open the pelvic floor. Apply root lock to open the low back and deepen into the fold.

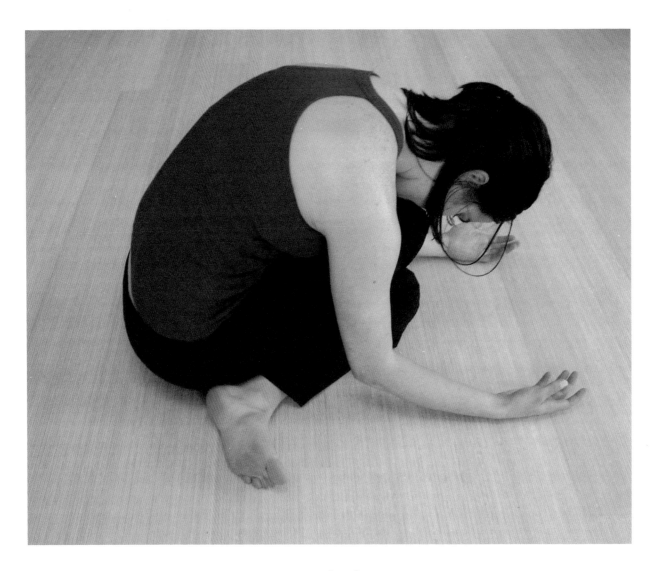

pose: shoelace

Sit cross-legged and draw the top right knee toward the midline. Draw the left bottom knee toward the midline until the knees are stacked as close as possible. Come into a forward fold. Feel the sensation of lengthening tension deep in the posterior right hip and the low back. There will also be sensation in the upper back and neck. If the sensation behind the neck is too much, lift the head from time to time and then come back into the fold.

Apply neck lock to lengthen the spine and release the back of the neck. Apply root lock to open the low back and deepen into the fold in shoelace and full butterfly.

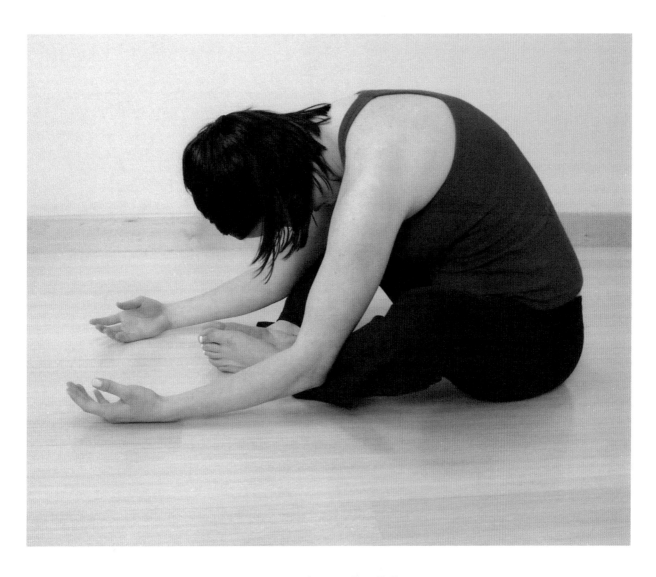

pose: butterfly, full

Sit with the soles of the feet together, two hand lengths away from the inner groin. Pull on the shins and come fully erect to begin. If you are unable to fully extend the spine, prop the hips on a folded blanket or pillow. Once you are extended, drop the head, round the shoulders and allow the window of the low back to open. Feel the lengthening tension in the full spine and inner groin. Keep the arms relaxed. If there is beyond the edge tension in the back of the neck, lift the head from time to time then resume the fold.

target: legs

release: pokey ball, thigh

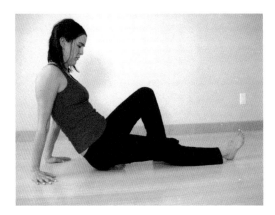

Sit with the right leg extended and place the pokey ball just distal to the sit bone. Allow your body weight to release this area, massaging all the way down to the back of the knee joint. Pause at any particularly tight areas to breathe and let go.

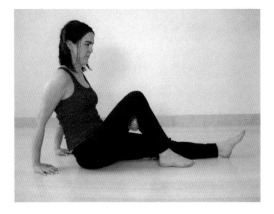

End this session on the posterior thigh by squeezing the ball nestled behind the knee, between the lower thigh and the upper calf.

For both back of the thigh poses, use this breath and bhanda focus: apply neck lock to lengthen the spine. Apply root lock to stabilize the low back and deepen into the lengthening sensation behind the thigh.

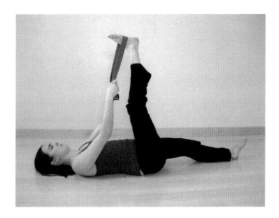

pose: thigh, strap

Lay on back, hips and knees bent, feet flat on floor. Place a strap above the heel in the arch of the right foot. Hold the strap as close to the foot as possible, elbows extended, shoulders relaxed. Feel the sensation of lengthening tension in the posterior thigh. To create more of a tension edge, extend the left leg to the floor and/or draw the right toes toward the face.

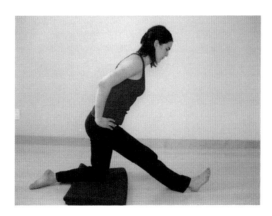

pose: thigh, kneeling

Kneel on a soft blanket. Keeping hips level, extend the right leg, heel on the floor, toes straight up. Feel the sensation of lengthening tension in the posterior thigh. Keep the spine straight, heart center lifted and angle forward only at the hip joint.

target: low back, hips & legs

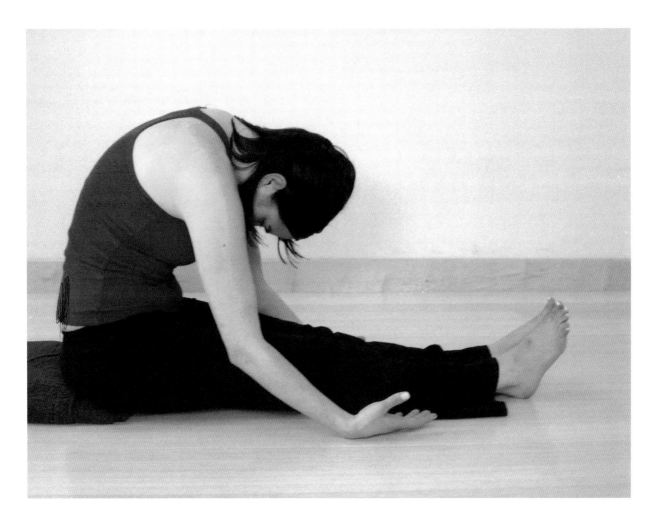

pose: caterpillar

Sit with legs extended, knees facing up. If you are unable to fully extend the spine perpendicular to the ground, prop the hips on a folded blanket or pillow. Once you are extended, drop the head, round the shoulders and allow the window of the low back to open. Feel the sensation of lengthening tension in the full spine, posterior hip and posterior thigh. If the sensation in the neck is too intense, lift the head from time to time then resume the fold. Try anchoring the upturned palms under the thighs, knees or calves.

Apply neck lock to lengthen the spine and deepen the sensation in the back of the neck. Apply root lock to open the low back and deepen into the fold.

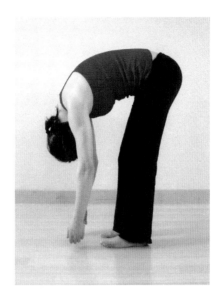

pose: forward fold, standing

Stand with the feet hip width apart, straight knees. Come into a forward fold by releasing the head, shoulders and low back, pouring the spine out of the pelvis.

Increase the sensation of lengthening tension in these areas by:

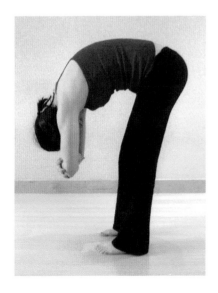

cradling the elbows in the hands

or

supporting the upper back on the wall.

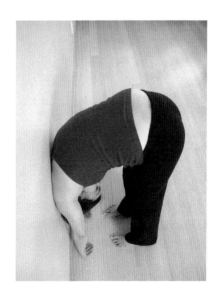

Apply neck lock to lengthen the spine. Apply root lock to open the low back and deepen into the fold.

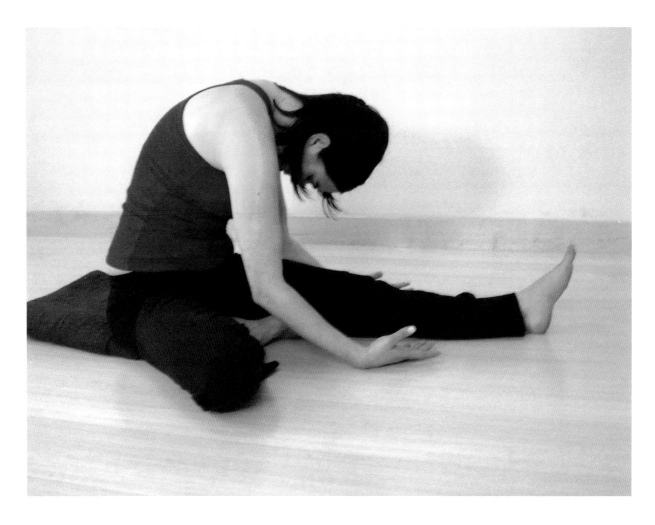

pose: butterfly, half

Sit with the left leg fully extended and the right foot positioned against the left inner thigh. If you are unable to fully extend the spine, prop the hips on a folded blanket or pillow. Once you are extended, turn the belly and chest toward the left leg. Drop the head, round the shoulders and allow the window of the low back to open. Deepen the left hip crease, coming into the fold at the hip joint. Feel the sensation of lengthening tension in the full spine, right side waist and posterior hip, and left posterior thigh. Keep the arms relaxed. If sensation is too intense in any part of the spine, lift the head from time to time then resume the fold.

Apply neck lock to lengthen the spine. Apply root lock to open the low back and deepen into the lengthening sensation behind the thigh.

Brought to my Knees

This morning I am brought to my knees
by a few simple lines from the Ashtavakra Gita:

"All things arise,
suffer change,
and pass away.
This is their nature.
When you know this
…you become still.
It is easy."

Excuse me? I have accumulated
sizable heaps of suffering evidence:
rampant ambition and dogged addiction,
messy relationships and hoards of stuff.
Pride shamelessly swaggers round
the whole sorry pile.

All this folly occurs in the context
of one breath following the next,
in a body eager to investigate
the nature of resistance, the quality of longing,
how it feels to turn away. Devoted
to the practice of mindfulness, surrender,
forgiveness, loving kindness.

Still there are long moments,
hours, whole days besmirched
with careless distraction.

Yet in this morning stillness
there is clear radiant allowance,
ample space for my twisted delivery to truth
brought to light in the way humans do it.

bella

pose: dragonfly, 3 variations:

Sit with legs as wide apart as possible, extended in front of you. If you are unable to fully extend the spine perpendicular to the ground, prop the hips on a folded blanket or pillow. Once you are extended, drop the head, round the shoulders and allow the window of the low back to open.

Apply neck lock to lengthen the spine and the back of the neck. Apply root lock to open the low back and deepen into the lengthening sensation behind the thigh and the inner groins.

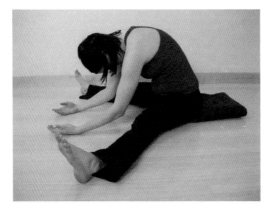

center dragonfly: Fold down between the legs. Feel the sensation of lengthening tension in the full spine, groin, posterior hips and posterior thighs.

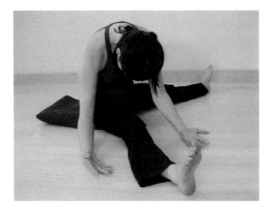

twisted dragonfly: Turn the belly and chest toward the right leg and fold down over the right leg. Feel the sensation of lengthening tension in the full spine, groin, left side waist, right posterior hip and both posterior thighs.

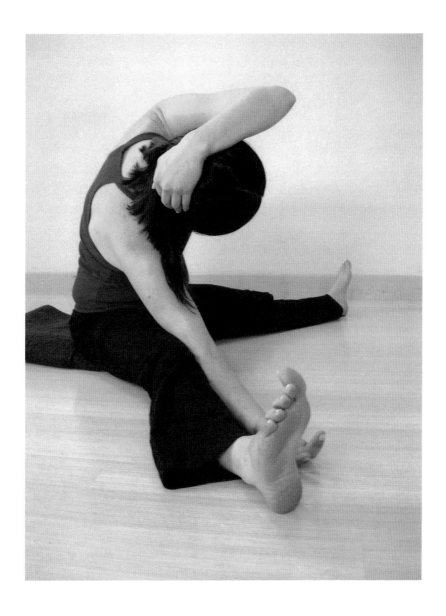

side bend dragonfly: Stretch the right arm along the inside or the top of the right leg, maintaining a side bend of the spine, without folding forward. Reach up with the left arm, turn the palm to the right and bring the upper arm as close to the left ear as possible. Bend the elbow and let the arm rest on the head. Feel the sensation of lengthening tension in the full spine, groin, left side waist and rib cage, right posterior hip and both posterior thighs. Keep the arms relaxed. If this is too much sensation in the neck, lift the head from time to time then resume the fold.

target: ankles & feet

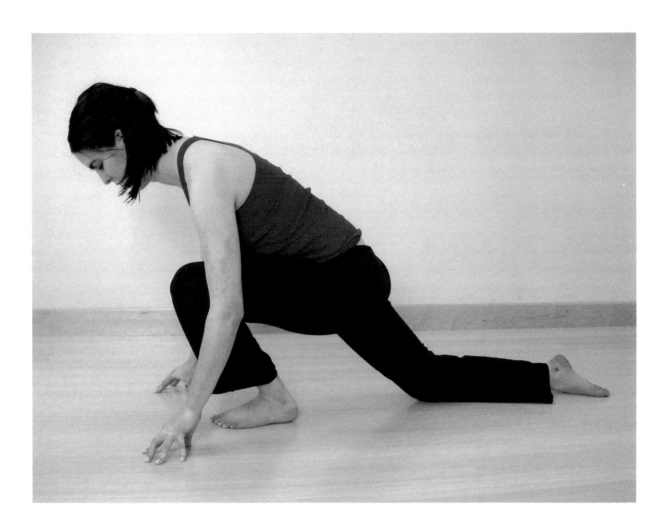

pose: lunge, heel cord

Come into lunge with left knee bent enough so it is positioned in front of the ankle, hands resting on the floor in front of the foot. Allow the belly and/or chest to rest on the top of the left thigh. Feel the sensation of lengthening tension in the left calf all the way down to the heel. Scoot the right leg back until you feel the matching sensation of lengthening tension in front of the right hip.

Apply neck lock to lengthen the full spine. Apply root lock to stabilize the low back and increase sensation in front hip of the leg that is extended back.

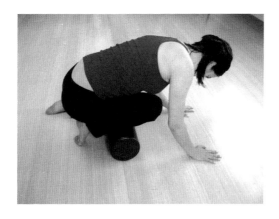

release: foam roller, shins

Come into child's pose with the shin on the roller, balancing with your hands on the floor in front. Shift the hips to the right and massage the outer shin, pausing at any areas of tension to breathe and release.

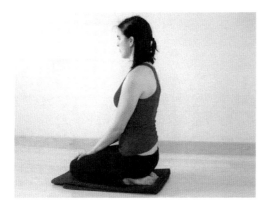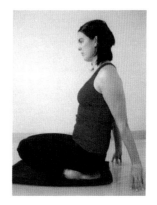

pose: foot, ankle instep

Come into seated rock pose, hips resting on heels. Keep the heart center lifted. This may be enough tension in front of the ankle for some and if it is too much, roll a towel to place under the ankle. Create a sensation of lengthening tension across the front of the ankle.

To increase the sensation, lean back on the hands keeping the heart lifted, slowly raising the knees. Graduate to resting the hands on the upraised thighs.

release: foot, self massage

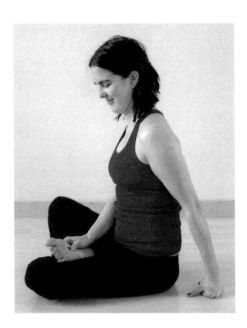

Sit cross legged and use the thumb to create parallel massage sweeps from the edge of the heel to the base of the toes. This is the plantar fascia and tight nodular areas are not normal. Dig into these areas to release.

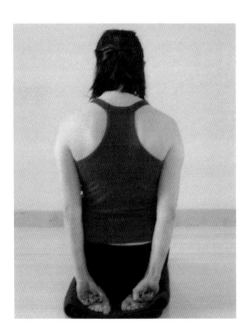

Come into seated rock pose, hips resting on heels. Use the knuckles on both soles at once to sweep from the base of the toes to the heel and back, searching again for tight nodular areas.

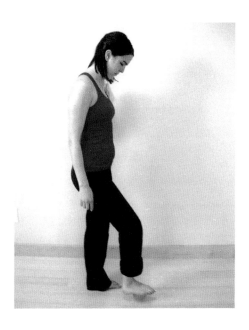

release: pokey ball, foot

Stand balancing on the left leg and place the sole of the right foot on the ball. Massage the area between the ball of the foot and the heel, digging into tight nodular areas. Come to a deeper edge of sensation by putting more of your body weight on to the pokey ball.

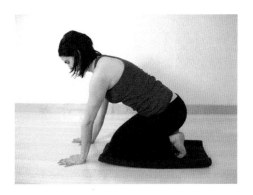 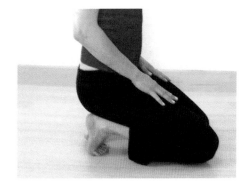

pose: foot squat

Come to hands and knees and curl toes under. Give extra encouragement to the baby toe which always loves to escape! Increase the sensation of lengthening tension at the base of the toes and the arch by bringing more weight back toward the hips. A soft blanket under the knees and toes will decrease the tension. When you are ready, come to full seated rock pose, toes curled under. Anchor attention in breath and sensation.

relaxation

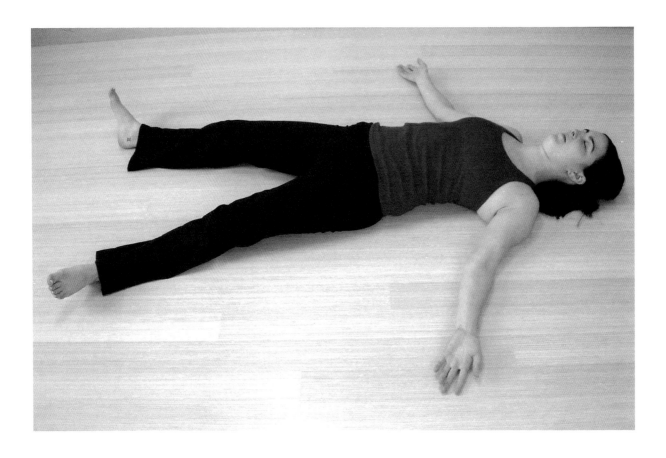

shivasana

Complete your session with this final pose. It is great practice to rest for a short while, allowing all that you have done to integrate and settle. Lay on your back and create what your body needs for comfort and full surrender to gravity. Spend the first minute making adjustments tracking and releasing any felt sense of tension. Once you are comfortable, commit to stillness in the body. Let that stillness anchor your attention to the quiet of your breathing and any physical sensation you notice. Let these anchors continue to support a practice of mindful meditation.

practice possibilities

Connective tissue change happens when stresses are applied with consistent practice. Choose one pose and practice it for five minutes most days and you will see changes within a month. The time you choose to devote to practice does not have to be the same each day nor do you have to do the same sequences. Ask your body what it needs. These techniques are a great way to warm up or cool down to other more vigorous activities. Many of the yin poses can be done with the soft propping available in a warm bed when you first wake or before going to sleep.

If possible, use the balls and roller on your special places before the poses. I like to at least release the spine with the tennis balls or roller and roller release the side leg. Here are a few possible yin sequences to follow. Build slowly to five minutes in each pose. Use these ideas for lift off. Cultivate listening to your body so you can hear what it needs. This is the essence of becoming your own best body worker.

3 beginner sequences:
- sphinx, caterpillar, twist to each side
- butterfly, sphinx, twist to each side
- child, lunge, twist to each side

intermediate sequence:
- butterfly, dragonfly, lunge, seal, saddle, child, twist to each side

preparatory sequences for:

half saddle or saddle:
instep ankle, side quad, lunge, sphinx, saddle, child, twist to each side

dragonfly:
happy baby, frog or wide legs up the wall, shoe lace, caterpillar, butterfly, dragonfly, twist to each side

snail:
butterfly, ½ butterfly, happy baby, passive neck hang, snail, sphinx, twist to each side

nervous system

Angel Wing and Breathing with Pelvic Motion are neural tension techniques. They are included in this manual as physical therapy treatment for clients with nervous system involvement. It is best to seek the service of a qualified professional if you have pain, numbness or tingling in the arms or legs.

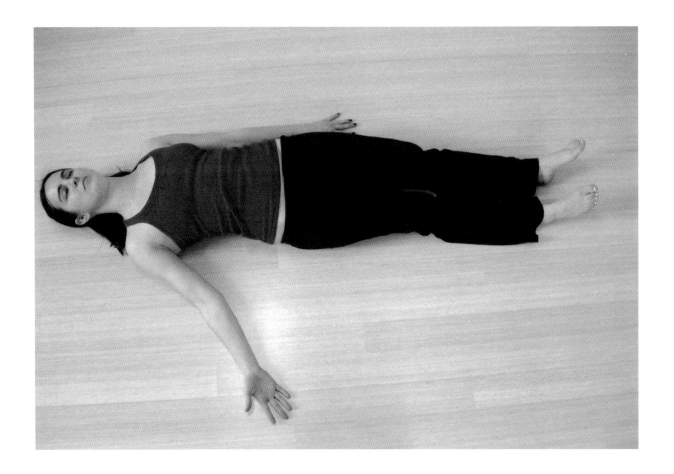

angel wing

Lay on your back, legs extended, arms palm down at your side. You are searching for the first experience of any tension in the arm. Turn the palm slowly up and see if that creates tension in the forearm or shoulder. If it does, stop there. If it does not, slowly slide the arm along the floor and stop when you feel the first tension sign. Remember this angle of the shoulder. You will use this self test before and after releases and poses.

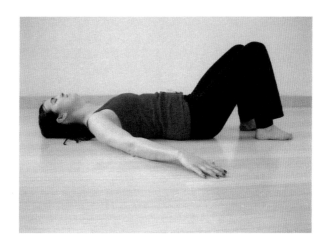

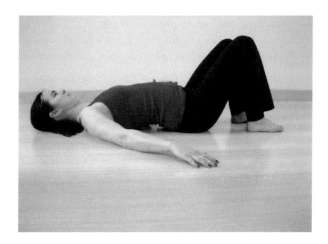

breathing with pelvic motion

Lay with hips and knees bent, feet flat on the floor. Exhale and flatten your low back toward the floor. Inhale and gently arch your back. Complete the motion smoothly and gently, working in an entirely pain free range. Observe the natural accompanying motion of your neck. With no effort on your part, the neck curve flattens as you arch your low back. Often the neck curve increases and your chin gently lifts as you flatten your low back.

When there is ease with this motion, try these two variations. 1) Position arms out to side, palms up on the inhale, down on the exhale. 2) Inhale, releasing knees to one side, turning head the opposite way. Exhale back to center. Turn the palm up on the side you are looking toward, down on the other sde. Change with the breath. Make it a perfect marriage of breath and motion.

Commitment

My hands and feet had a conversation today
overheard by my hips and heart
who had their own private tete-a-tete.

Soon my heart spoke directly to my hands,
which spurned my hips to inquire about my feet.

My tail wiggled its way up my spine
landing at the pinnacle of my head
and my face broke into a spacious grin.

I showed up big time, electrified
by the chance encounter with another,
torching the field with an aliveness
that threw wide my heart,
ecstasy spilling onto the sidewalk,
so absorbed that my rambling mind
succumbed to emptiness.

And with just a little extra time and space
the muffled longing of my soul got a foothold,
carved out some juicy territory
and summoned my spirit to hover in the room,
a stranger no more.

bella

core stability

Tune into your breath and activate your bhandas to stabilize your core. We can do this as formal exercise and we can also utilize many random moments during the day to turn our awareness to stability: walking, stairs, lifting, getting up and down from sitting, you name it! Turning on the bhandas during the warm up phase of any exercise will activate them and afford you protection as you begin to move more vigorously, especially if you have done some release work in tight areas first.

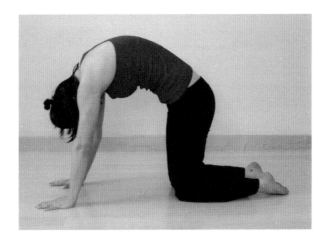

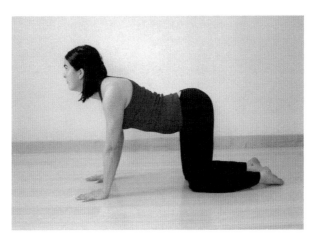

cat cow

Find a neutral table top position with the knees directly under the hips and the hands beneath the shoulders. Exhale and apply root lock to drop the tail and head toward the floor and round the spine to the ceiling. Inhale to release the pelvic floor open and lift the tail bone and head toward the ceiling. Allow the spine to completely sag into an arch.

core abs

Use this breath & bhanda pattern in each of the following exercises: exhale and apply root lock as you move into the challenge of the stability. Inhale back to the starting position. Do not let the arch in the lumbar spine increase or decrease.

Start with just the hips and knees bent, feet on the floor and try the breath and bhanda pattern. Then increase the difficulty with this progression:

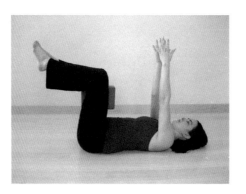

lifting one leg @ a time — opposite hip does not move

Bend knees and hips at right angles, calves parallel to the floor, arms pointing straight up, palms toward each other. Root lock on the exhale, release the lock on the inhale. Add a yoga block between the thighs to squeeze on the exhale, release the squeeze on the inhale. Each exhale is a chance to re-commit to root lock.

Progress by exhaling one or both arms over head and/or, extend the legs out from the center. Do not let the arch in the lumbar spine increase or decrease.

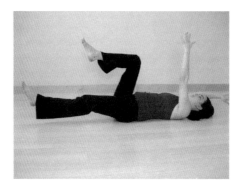

Increase the challenge by removing the block and exhaling the opposite arm and leg out and/or both arms and legs out.

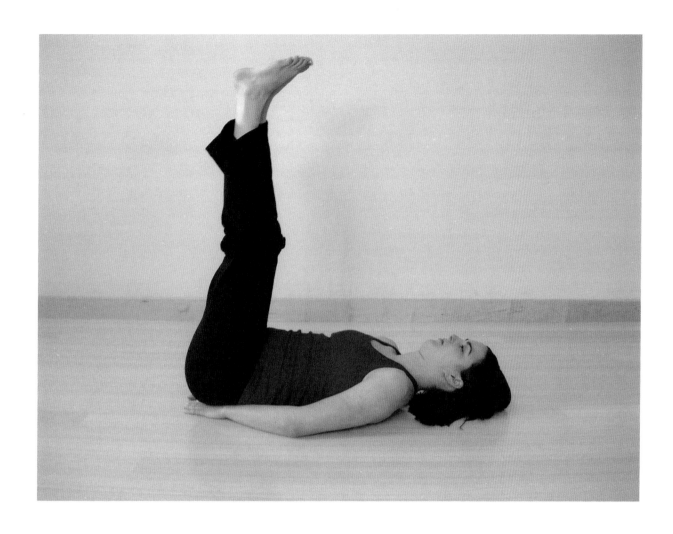

Place hands under sacrum for support, legs straight up. Exhale, apply root lock and lower the legs toward the floor. Do not let the arch in the lumbar spine increase or decrease. Hold the legs hovering above the floor for several breaths or inhale legs up and exhale them down. Recommit to the root lock with each exhale. Use an exhale to draw knees to chest and relax.

core hips

Lay on back, hips and knees bent, feet on the floor under the knees. Inhale and raise the hips off the floor. Exhale and apply root lock, maintaining the position of the hips off the floor. Stay up through several breaths, recommitting to the root lock on the exhale.

Increase the difficulty with this progression:

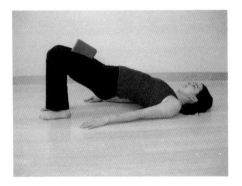

Add a yoga block between the thighs. Exhale, squeeze the block and apply root lock as you raise the hips. Inhale and release all the way to the floor.

Increase the challenge by staying up through several breaths, using the exhale to re-commit to root lock.

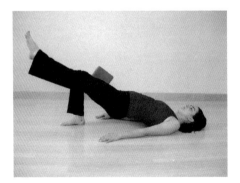

Increase the challenge further by using each exhale to extend one leg parallel to the floor. Feel the hip on the other side working hard to keep the pelvis stable. Inhale to return foot to the starting position on the ground. Continue, letting the breath pace the motion of alternating leg extensions.

"Meditation is like training a puppy, you say 'stay' but after a few breaths, the puppy wanders away. You go back and gently pick it up and bring it back."

Jack Kornfield

Stillness Mat

She never really changes,
always drooling at the door,
just the slimmest temptation,
bolt eager for a leap into the wild.

A tender tug on the leash,
reigns this seasoned puppy in,
guides her back to obedience
on the stillness mat.

But then, the other day,
an inspired thunderbolt:
after twenty years,
this ain't no puppy!

This dog is friggin' old,
arthritis in both hips, random
grey whiskers jut askew from her
canine yellow maw.

Weepy-eyed by the door,
listless panting,
she doesn't really want to go out
but dogged habits die hard.

I lay down beside her,
my cheek on fleecy flanks
and weep for mercy.
I don't want to go either.

Together we lay
on the stillness mat,
track the persistent parade
streaming right by without us.

bella

mountain pose

We can practice core stability and gain a sense of deep internal support while standing. This is an exercise that can be practiced frequently during the most random moments of the day: standing in line, walking, doing housework. Functional practice builds a strong core and will eventually shift your alignment in healthy ways. Interrupt this practice frequently and let go of all effort, relaxing into your natural standing posture.

• Swing the heels out a little bit so the outer borders of the feet are parallel. Equalize the weight across the ball of the foot from the big toe side to the little toe side. Now equalize the weight between the ball of the foot and a mid point on the heel.

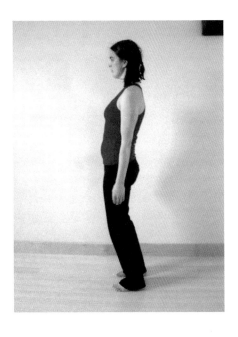 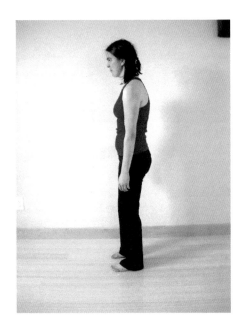

Notice the increased weight on the ball of the foot, the over arched low back and caved in chest.

Notice the increased weight on the heel, the flattened low back and rounded shoulders.

Feel the subtle possibility that you may be putting more of your weight on the right or left foot. If this is true, shift the contents of the belly over to the light side to equalize the weight on both feet.

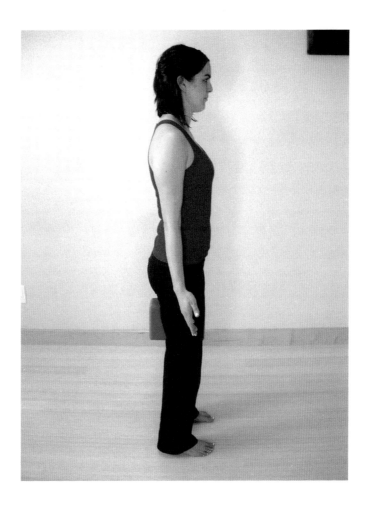

• Exhale and recruit the inner thigh muscles as if you are squeezing a yoga block. Feel the aliveness of the inner thigh muscles. Try drawing the knee caps gently up into the thighs to increase this sense of aliveness.

• Gently draw the pelvic floor up and in; lightly draw the deep abdominals to the back body. Imagine a big smile suspended across the front of the hip bones. Unclench the buttocks.

• Inhale and gently lift the chest away from the hips. Lengthen the back of neck and roll the tops of the ears slightly forward.

• Feel the shoulder blades melt down the back body, inviting the palms a little forward in the room.

• Keep the breath coming continuously. Exhale and feel the rooted connection from the deep belly, pelvic floor, inner thigh and feet into the earth. Inhale and lengthen upward, lifting the heart center away from the belly and lengthening the back of the neck.

the real world

lifting

From a solid sense of mountain pose, we can learn how to lift safely. A young, healthy body with a good spine can generally lift up to 20#, bending and twisting in ways that do not work when the weight is heavier or the body not so young and pliable.

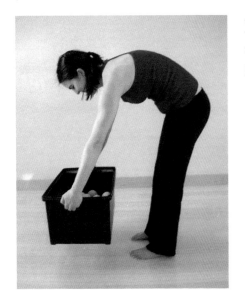

Lifting with a rounded back, especially when we add a twist, is one of the many ways we unconsciously create injuries.

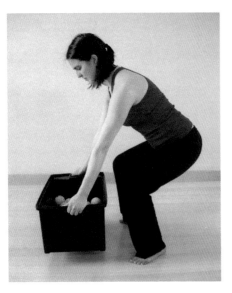

Use a wide stance and keep the back straight from the sacrum to the crown. Lean forward from the hip joint, not the low back. Apply root and neck lock as you straighten the legs and feel the extra power delivered through the bhandas.

sitting

It is hard to know what the human body can ideally bear, but we definitely were not designed to sit all day, even in the best of chairs. It would be great if we could take a break from sitting every 20-30 minutes and limit the total number of hours we sit each day. Evaluate where you spend the most time sitting each day and do what is possible to come into neutral alignment with or without support.

Even with the best intentions, here is how so many of us look after awhile.

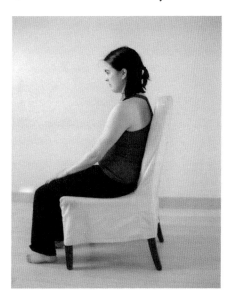

Sometimes perching at the edge of the chair is the best option. Use a support for the lumbar spine if needed. The spinal curves are much happier when established at neutral with the head resting over the shoulders, the back of the neck long. Have the feet flat on the floor, the knees a little lower than the hips.

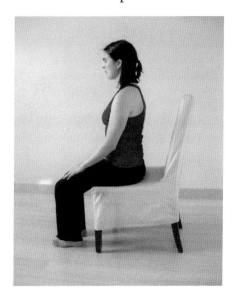

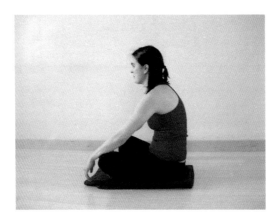

When it's time to sit on the floor or do yoga it is even harder to hold a neutral spine. The most challenging seated position is cross legged. In this picture, the low back and upper back are rounded. The neck is over extended with the chin poking forward. When the knees are higher than the hips it is almost impossible to have a neutral aligned spine.

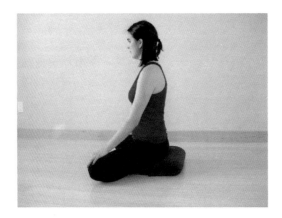

Prop the hips on just the right amount of blanket, pillow or zafu to create the possibility of neutral. The ideal height creates a gentle amount of effort to maintain a curve in the low back. Lift the heart center and let the head rest over the body. It is possible to have too much low back arch. Many people tilt the pelvis too far forward and over extend the low back. Finding the middle ground is our calling. Cross legged sitting is inherently an asymmetrical pose. Change the cross of the legs from time to time.

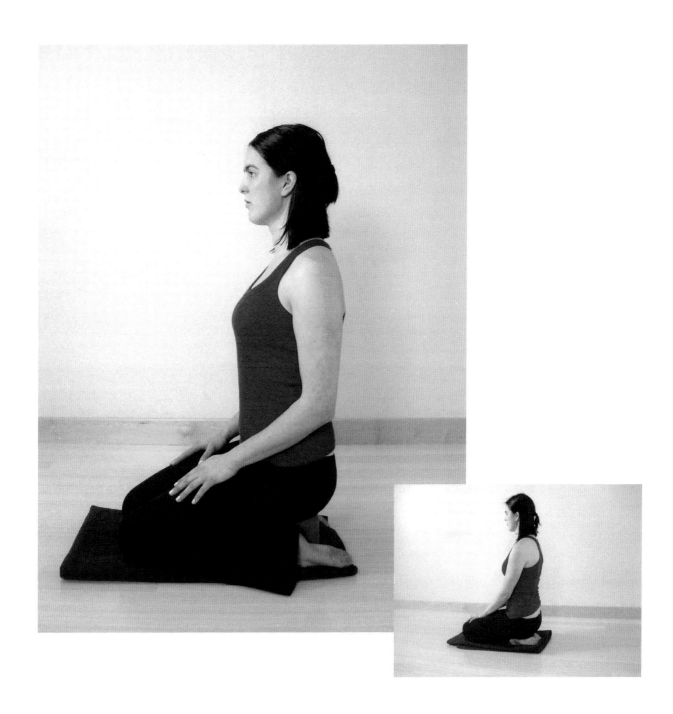

Seated rock pose is a symmetrical seated pose and a good alternative to sitting cross legged. In the full expression of this pose, the hips rest on the ground between the feet. For less tension in the front of the thighs, sit on the heels or place a yoga block under the sit bones. Establishing the low back curve becomes easier here when the hips are higher than the knees. Feel the heart center and head fall into place above the hips.

Sanctuary

I take a refuge in wisdom that
speaks of awakening,
sings tall tales of freedom,
power points the possible,
not for others only,
but sure-fire faith
in my own eternal spiral landing
into a true blue nature:
the unchained body-heart
exposed over a temporal lifetime.

I take a refuge in teachings that
dance at my feet,
pierce my heart,
liberate my mind,
all the ancient commandments
and all that is breath taking fresh:
wake up calls that relentlessly ring,
random episodes that dash
my rampant illusions,
respites in the lap of nature
that grant resolve to abide
recurrent heartbreak.

And I take a refuge in community,
reality journey companions,
the back up bunch,
each waking to our own
vulnerable drummer
in our own sweet time,
sweet touch of pliant bodies unearthed,
pressed by hearts made public,
minds loosening to the same beat.

I take a refuge.

bella

conclusion

If you have worked your way through this guide on your own, consider yourself introduced to basic concepts used in individual physical therapy sessions and yoga classes. Whether you have explored this territory independently or in a group class, an individual session will guide you toward a more specific approach for your unique body and its particular constellation of challenges.

Whether you need help getting started or can use this guide independently, we can all learn to be our own best body worker. Increased symptoms brought on by any of these exercises is never a healthy sign. Practice 100% mindfulness by being in full relationship with your aches and pains. Be gentle and move only in ways that feel healing for your body.

Congratulations on embarking on a rich healing journey toward more full embodiment. I share this lifetime of learning in the hope that you will enjoy this opportunity to be playful, be creative, be intuitive and test my favorite maxim from my teacher, Gabrielle Roth:

"It takes discipline to be a free spirit."

Many blessings on your own unique journey toward freedom.

just for you

index

Made in the USA
Charleston, SC
06 March 2012